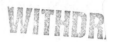

Medicine

Questions and answers

with full explanations

Sri Hari Ravi
Amisha Patel
Veena Babu

Sri Hari Ravi, Amisha Patel and Veena Babu

ISBN-13: **978-1481830386**

ISBN-10: **1481830384**

DEDICATION

I have too many people to thank in helping me put this

resource together.

My mum, Bharath, Aathi, Vee, Shiv, Jas and Neal, to

name a few.

I hope this books accomplishes its goal of helping you

in fulfilling your ambitions and getting your place in

medical school.

Hari

CONTENTS

Medical Based Questions

1. What do you understand about how cancer is formed?

2. How can the risk of heart attack be reduced?

3. How does smoking increase the risk of cancer and cardiovascular disease?

4. What have you recently read about the role of genetics in medicine?

5. Do you think bowel cancer is common in the UK? Explain your answer.

6. What can be done to help prevent cervical cancer?

7. How does MRI work?

8. How does Ultrasound imaging work?

9. What is the structure of DNA?

10. What is Down's syndrome?

11. What are the differences between diseases in developing countries and those faced in the UK?

12. Where are cholera and typhoid found and what are their symptoms?

13. What is the most common genetic disorder in the UK?

14. Can you describe how Down's syndrome would manifest in a child?

15. Which piece of imaging equipment do you consider to be the most important?

16. Why are x-rays potentially dangerous?

17. Describe the process of fertilisation.

18. Why is there no vaccination for the common cold?

19. What problems are caused by obesity?

20. Name an antibiotic.

21. Why do scars form from wounds?

22. What is a retrovirus?

23. Describe the transmission of an impulse across a synapse.

24. What is an ECG?

25. What is herd immunity?

26. Describe the problems with embryonic stem cells.

Ethical Based Questions

1. If you were given £100,000 to spend on a developing country, how would you use it?

2. Is death acceptable for a Jehovah's witness if they refuse a blood transfusion?

3. If, on a scale of 0 to 5, 0 was caring for people and 5 was an interest in science, where would you put yourself on the scale?

4. Would you feel emotionally affected if a patient died?

5. Why do you consider the suicide rate in doctors is high?

6. What do you think of stem cell research and the possibility of using it to treat diabetes?

7. Would you empathise or sympathise?

8. Would you think that you have failed if one of your patients died?

9. Can you name the four ethical principles of medicine?

10. Do you believe an alcoholic has the same right as a non-alcoholic to receive treatment and potentially a transplant?

11. Do you believe euthanasia is acceptable? Explain your answer.

12. Do you think those who have physical disabilities should be allowed to practice medicine?

13. Is it fair for the NHS to dedicate time and resources to patients who have self-inflicted conditions?

14. Would you operate on an obese person despite knowing that the operation's effects may be void in 6 months for example with a hip replacement?

15. Is it okay for doctors to experience personal feelings towards their patients?

16. Do you think doctors should have the right to strike?

17. What are the arguments for and against a ban on selling tobacco?

18. What is more important; quality of life or length of life?

19. What are the arguments for and against abortion?

20. What is the importance of learning about ethics?

21. What are the advantages and disadvantages of a private health care system?

22. Should the HPV vaccine be available on the NHS?

Why did you choose to apply for Medicine at this particular university?

1. Tell me about yourself and something interesting you have done?

2. What can you contribute to this university?

3. What do you know about the way we teach medicine?

4. What do you know about the different medical degree programmes?

5. What do you know about intercalated BSc?

6. If you like the systems based course, why did you apply to Cambridge?

7. Explain your choices of university on your UCAS form.

8. What extra-curricular activities would you consider joining here if you were offered a place?

9. What are you going to do for us, without mentioning your academic achievements?

10. You said you like the course structure here, how do you think the Systems and Topics based structure here is going to help the future of Medicine?

11. What are the qualities about our medical school attract you the least?

12. What do you know about PBL? Why do you want to come to a PBL medical school?

Personal qualities about you based questions

1. What makes you a good doctor?

2. Take us through your personal statement?

3. How did you prepare for this interview?

4. What qualities make a poor doctor?

5. How has your journey been thus far?

6. Do you eat healthily?

7. Do you have any family in the medical profession, if so have they influenced you in any way to become a doctor?

8. What do you do to relax?

9. Sell yourself to us for 2 minutes?

10. Do you read? What was the last book you read?

11. What genre of films or books are you most interested in?

12. Are you a people person or do you prefer to be alone?

13. Do you enjoy working in a team?

14. Have you ever experienced death?

15. Medicine is a very long and stressful subject to study, how do you currently deal with stress?

16. Tell me about any of the situations where you have shown leadership skills.

17. In ten years' time after you have become a doctor and all your friends want to have a reunion but you are unable to attend, how would you want them to remember you?

18. What are the most important attributes for maintaining good working relationship between colleagues?

19. Do you do anything that involves working in a team?

20. How can you relate being a doctor to playing competitive sport?

21. Have you ever considered taking a gap year?

22. Give examples of where you have used teamwork and leadership skills?

23. What did you do for Duke of Edinburgh?

24. Have you ever had to make an unpopular decision as a leader?

25. Do you believe your communication and organisational skills are adequate to become a great doctor?

26. What do you do in your spare time?

27. What would you describe as your worst qualities?

28. How would your closest friends describe you?

29. How do you handle criticism?

30. Give me an example when you have had your opinions overridden, what did you do?

31. What is your ten year plan?

32. What person(s) has had the biggest positive impact on you?

33. How have you developed your communication skills?

Work experience and education based questions

1. How are your A-levels going?

2. How would any non-science subject at GCSE/A-level help as a doctor?

3. Out of the non-science subjects that you have studied, which one do you think will be useful in career in medicine and why?

4. Out of the work experience you have done, what did you enjoy the most?

5. Tell us about your work experience?

6. Which of your work experience placements did you enjoy the most? What was your role there? Was it organised by your school?

7. What did you learn from your work experience?

8. Have you ever raised money for charity?

9. How do you contribute to the life of your school?

10. How would your headmaster describe you?

11. You seem to have a wide variety of work experience but seem to lack work experience at a GP's practice and in hospital. Have you done anything else which you have not mentioned?

12. You come from a college with 1500 people, do you find that daunting?

13. What do you currently contribute to your college?

14. What kind of voluntary work have you done, how has it helped you?

15. You visited nursing homes for the blind, what did you do there?

16.   What was the worst part of your work experience?

17.   Do you remember any particular patient that did not have a good outcome?

18.   Did you see any patients that had a good outcome?

19.   What steps have you taken to learn more about medicine?

20.   What is your greatest achievement you have attained thus far in your education?

21.   What in the history of medicine has really interested you?

22.   What impressed you most about the doctors in your work experience?

23.   Describe a difficult situation you have dealt with in your work experience and what did you learn from it?

24.   Have you ever been in a position of responsibility and something went wrong?

INDUSTRY BASED QUESTIONS

1. Do you think pharmacists are sometimes tempted to advise a customer to buy an expensive product even if there is a cheaper one available?

2. How will 'The Human Genome Project' help treat patients in the future?

3. What are the advantages and disadvantages to 'The Human Genome Project'?

4. What sort of laws should be passed on to prevent people taking advantages over 'The Human Genome Project'?

5. Have there been any dramatic changes to the NHS since it was founded?

6. Did you know your local health authority has the largest number of bed blockers? How should the NHS go about removing bed blockers?

7. What is wrong with the NHS?

8. What does the World Health Organisation do?

9. If you were the head of a group of doctors and a colleague was not doing the job well, what would you do?

10. If you were asked to design four stamps to mark the 50th anniversary of the NHS, what would you put on the stamps and why?

11. If you where the prime minister what three government policies would you set to achieve?

12. Give me three extended roles of nurses in the modern healthcare system?

13. How do you think the health system should be funded? Give me your opinion.

14. European Working Directive - what do you know about them?

15. What do you believe should be the uniform for doctors in these modern times?

16. Is the Hippocratic Oath still relevant today?

17. Who are the General Medical Council?

18. Who are the Medicines and Healthcare products Regulatory Agency (MHRA)?

19. What is holistic medicine?

20. **In your opinion, where do you see the health service going?**

21. Do you read newspapers? Name an interesting medical related story.

22. How do you go about keeping up-to-date with current medical issues?

23. **What do you read of a medical nature?**

24. Tell us about any medical articles you have seen in the media recently?

25. What do you believe has been the biggest recent breakthrough in medicine?

26. What was the last book/article you read about medicine?

27. What major issues are currently affecting the NHS?

28. How do you think doctors are viewed in the current media?

29. What do you consider to be important advances in medicine over the last 50 years?

30. How do you think the rise in technology has influenced and will continue to influence the practice of medicine?

31. What social factors can affect people seeking medical help?

32. What is the role of the minister of health?

Your view on becoming a doctor based questions

1.What is your impression of the job of a doctor?

2.Do you think doctors just work from 9am- 5pm?

3.What do you think most people who qualify in medicine do?

4.Have you ever considered becoming a G.P.?

5.What are the positive and negative aspects about being a doctor?

6.Would you like to be a nurse?

7.Do you think a doctor's job is stressful?

8.If you did not get a place to study medicine, what other profession would you be interested in?

9.What makes a good team member?

10. What qualities does a doctor need?

11. A banker works long hours, why are they different from a doctor?

NHS Changes 2013 based questions

1. Can patients receive any treatment they want under the NHS?

2. If the NHS is funded by taxation and patients need to pay for dental treatment, what happens to those patients who are not currently being taxed?

3. On your application I can see that you did some work experience in a GP clinic and on an acute ward in a hospital. What differences did you observe and which did you prefer?

4. Can you give an example of any recent unsuccessful ventures undertaken by the NHS? Why do you think it was unsuccessful?

5. Can you give an example of any projects undertaken by the NHS that have been a success?

6. Do you know of any upcoming advances in healthcare that the NHS is supporting?

7. What do you know about the General Medical Council?

8. Do you know the purpose of the British Medical Association?

9. If you could change one thing about the NHS what would it be and why?

General points to consider

The interview

The interview process differs between medical schools and you may be called for an interview any time between November and April. There is usually a panel of 2 or more interviewers and you may be given a scenario beforehand in the form of an article to read or a video to watch. The duration of the interview may last 20 minutes or more, however, the length is not a measure of success. Make sure you arrive early, as a combination of nerves and being late may cause you to panic. Avoid delays by planning ahead; this can be calculated by adding 20 minutes onto the maximum anticipated delay for your journey. Do your research on university parking facilities if you are travelling by car, or tube/train line suspensions and delays. In the unlikely event that you are late (after taking all the above measures), call the medical school as soon as you can and inform them of your anticipated arrival time.

For information on what to bring to the interview, consult your invitation letter from the university. A portfolio of achievements may be required by some medical schools, however, if it is not specified be prepared with the following:

- Tissues

- Water

- Reading material e.g. your personal statement, university brochure, health journal, campus map

- Supportive family member/teacher/friend or no-one if another person is too distracting (you will be interviewed alone!)

Preparation

It is important that you prepare for your interview as it can save you or be your downfall. Make sure that you find a balance between being under-prepared and being over-prepared, as both of these can lead to poor interview.

Clues to interviewers that you are under-prepared - if you have no idea what questions you may be asked, if you do not know what the NHS stands for, and if you do not know about any health related current affair topics. Clues to interviewers that you are over-prepared include - if you appear over-rehearsed and robotic such as being able to recite your answers word-perfect and without hesitation. Make sure give natural responses and expect the unexpected in regards to questions you will be asked, failure to do so can make you come across as too rigid and inflexible.

Use ethical terms appropriately when answering questions, the genuine consensus amongst interviewers is that inappropriate use of terminology often makes the candidate seem like they are trying too hard to be something they are not (in this case intelligent). Therefore, do not be too polished in your answers and be as natural as possible. The interview process will give you ample opportunity to highlight your strengths. Maturity can be demonstrated when you reflect on a question being asked by including your personal experience and achievements (make sure it is genuine).

Try and answer all questions in detail; see the wider picture and give your answers, putting the question into context, taking into account all situations/circumstances. Examples of how to do this are given consistently throughout the book. Emphasise your appreciation of complex questions, however, when presenting your answers be clear and concise. The use of good English is vitally important, so take your time when answering questions - you are expected to think carefully about questions before answering and not to roll answers off your tongue. Do not fall into the trap of answering questions instantaneously, you will be more likely to make a mistake with your grammar and once again it may appear unnatural.

When describing your personal qualities demonstrate a balance of confidence, intelligence and humility. Attempt not to sound cocky and only use your achievements as illustrative examples when answering questions. Remember the interviewers have read your personal statement and therefore you have already impressed them to a certain degree; the interview is an opportunity for them to find out more. Always provide examples where possible when answering questions about your achievements or capabilities, do not just talk in theory.

The use of non-verbal communication skills are also important and are vital to the doctor-patient relationship for building rapport. It is important that you display qualities such as honesty, trust, sincerity and modesty during your interview.

Be prepared for your personal statement to be scrutinised. Highlight the personal interests mentioned in your personal statement when asked about any aspect of it. When answering questions on why you want to become a doctor, be honest and show a realistic understanding of the role of a doctor, especially in relation to an area of medicine which you are particularly interested in for example paediatrics. Demonstrate a caring ability, but also provide clear reasons as to why you feel particularly drawn to becoming a doctor compared with other healthcare professions such as nursing.

Key points to consider:

- The detailed role and routine of a modern doctor

- Examples of how you have prepared for the interview

- Examples of how you have developed the qualities to become a doctor

- Enthusiasm, show that you want to find out more about a career in medicine. Remember there is no model answer for the question "why do you want to be a doctor?"

- Demonstrate a realistic perception that you know why a doctor is the only career for you.

Overcoming nerves

Being nervous is understandable, however, do not let it compromise your performance during the interview. The interviewers can tell if you are nervous by a trembling voice, unsettled hands and legs and blank mind. To overcome nerves, there are a number of techniques which can be put into practice:

- If you go blank, take a pause and think. This is far better than saying the first answer that comes into your head.

- Try to maintain a positive mental attitude

- Practice with someone intimidating

- Take some rescue remedy

  The night before your interview, re-read the necessary material such as your personal statement, current affairs articles, ethical dilemma articles and your BMAT essay. It is important to then relax, get some exercise, eat a light meal and get at least 8 hours of sleep.

Body Language

Body language represents a key part of the screening process for medical school. After viewing your personal statement and assessing your predicted grades, most universities will call those they are seriously considering of offering a place to for an interview. This will be your opportunity to put yourself on display and demonstrate why you are deserving of a place to study Medicine at their institution.

Body language incorporates many features. It includes the way you dress, act and react to questions during the interviewing process. It is therefore imperative to consider a few details regarding what is required of you when this time comes - it could make the difference on being denied a place or being offered a place at Medical School.

Do's + Don'ts

By studying medicine you will be required to meet members of the public on a daily basis.

The public want to be cared for by someone who they hold in high esteem and can be looked upon as a respected individual. Therefore, they **will** judge you even before you start to speak to them. One must therefore ensure that they are appropriately dressed and prepared. Denote the characteristics above in your appearance and behaviour so that the interviewer can be assured you meet the credentials of a future doctor. Shaking the interviewer's hand before you begin may highlight your professional manner and is advisable. Appear interested, approachable, relaxed and attentive. Try to naturally use the interviewers formal names e.g. Dr. Johnston, when answering or asking questions and note how they respond to you - this will make you look professional.

Body Posture

At all times maintain good posture with your back slightly relaxed but by avoiding slouching when walking and sitting down. Place both your hands together on your lap and avoid crossing your arms or fidgeting. Do not shy away from using your hands during dialogue, however, do this in moderation as it can become very distracting for the interviewer! As a woman, crossing your legs when wearing a skirt should be done to avoid embarrassment. Men should also attempt to cross their legs but keeping their legs moderately together is equally acceptable. Common postures which should be avoided are crossed arms, hands in pockets and slouching.

Gestures + Facial Expressions

By all means feel free to express yourself as this often emphasises how well you can communicate your thoughts and feelings to others; a good characteristic when working in a team. React well to jokes and good news with smiling and laughter but show concern and sadness when presented with less favourable information. The aim is to show that you can communicate in a manner appropriate to the situation (this should be no different to how you would react when talking to a friend!). For men, it is highly advisable to be clean shaven before the interview and to make sure your hair is neatly cut and not interfering with your face. For women, hair should be neatly tied or clipped back, away from your eyes and minimal makeup should be worn.

Eye Contact

This is vital when in conversation with the interviewer. Maintaining eye contact shows you can engage in conversation and not become easily distracted. It shows the interviewer that you are a confident individual and, most importantly, makes them feel comfortable talking and listening to you. This gives them an idea of how well you can engage with patients as a future medical student and indeed doctor.

This feature of body language is extremely important and should not be downplayed as it can easily lead to a poor interview if not executed well.

Clothing

For the interview in general men should wear a 2 piece clean suit with a tie and polished shoes. Avoid comedy ties and if you prefer not to wear a tie, make sure only the top button of your shirt is undone. Women have slightly more freedom in that they have a choice of a skirt or trousers with a blouse. A matching jacket can also be worn. Women should also wear polished shoes but avoid over-dressing, very high heels, cleavage, short or clingy skirts, patterned tights or stockings with holes. Do not feel afraid to showcase any badges from college/high school which highlight your current achievements (e.g. Prefect/ Head Boy badges), but keep this to a minimal.

Medical Based Questions

The key to answering a medical related question well is to take what may be a complex topic and present it clearly and simply. If you do not know the answer it is acceptable to let the interview panel know, however, medical based questions in this book should give you a rough idea of how to tackle the majority topics. We advise you to go away and thoroughly read any topic that comes up that you are not familiar with.

Patient.co.uk is a brilliant resource for answering medical questions in a clear way without using jargon. It's sometimes helpful to give a brief definition/overview of the condition as an introduction. If you are unsure, do not try and bluff your way through an answer as the examiner will see through it. Before answering any question, take a minute to think about it.

1. **What do you understand about how cancer is formed?**

"Cancer occurs when previously normal cells become abnormal and multiply uncontrollably at a faster rate than normal. This can lead to a cluster of abnormal cells called a tumour. The cancer can be classified as malignant, which is

when the tumor has invaded surrounding organs, or benign which does not invade other organs."

2. How can the risk of heart attack be reduced?

A heart attack is when part of the heart muscle dies, which means that the heart can no longer pump efficiently, leading to a reduction in the amount of blood passing via arteries around the body. The risk of a heart attack can be reduced by changing the way we live. Main changes include:

➢ *"Healthier diet: eat more fruit and vegetables, food that contains 'good' cholesterol and reduce fat intake.*

➢ *Stop smoking*

> ➤ *Take up exercise: 5 sessions of 30 minutes exercise each week. This should be vigorous enough to make you slightly out of breath.*

> ➤ *Lose weight if overweight or obese.*

> ➤ *Non-modifiable risk factors include gender, family history of heart disease, genetic abnormalities in cholesterol metabolism."*

3. How does smoking increase the risk of cancer and cardiovascular disease?

"Cigarettes contain cancer causing agents known as carcinogens, which can cause mutations (DNA errors) in cells. When cigarettes are smoked, carcinogens are released into the body and can eventually lead to cancer. The longer a person smokes the more carcinogens

they are exposed to; and therefore the higher the risk of cancer, especially lung cancer.

Smoking also causes narrowing of blood vessels, which increases the risk of an individual suffering from a stroke or a heart attack. The more an individual smokes, the narrower their vessels may become, increasing their risk of cardiovascular disease."

4. **What have you recently read about the role of genetics in medicine?**

In answering questions about research try and find a broad topic rather than a very niche topic. Discussing a broader topic shows that you are aware of the current issues and will be more able to answer questions on them.

"There has been a lot of work on looking at the effects of genetics on ageing, and scientists are trying to determine if particular genetic make-up makes you more susceptible to degenerative diseases such as Alzheimer's. Researchers at Kings College London have discovered biomarkers for Alzheimer's disease."

5. **Do you think bowel cancer is common in the UK? Explain your answer.**

Bowel cancer is the 3rd commonest cancer in the UK after lung and breast. Even if you do not know how common bowel cancer is you can use the answer to this question to demonstrate your knowledge of current medical issues. Over the last few years, bowel cancer screening in older individuals has increased in importance, highlighting that bowel cancer is an issue.

"I think that bowel cancer is a common issue in the UK, as medical literature (e.g. the BMJ and other medical journals), have been driving towards promoting bowel cancer screening, particularly in those aged over 65 years, as this leads to earlier diagnosis. In turn, this enables people to receive necessary treatment earlier, increasing the chances of complete recovery."

6. **What can be done to help prevent cervical cancer?**

This question is testing your knowledge of public health campaigns, in this case the HPV (human papilloma virus) vaccine and cervical smear testing.

"Cervical cancer is one of the commonest cancers occurring in women, but unfortunately is often detected too late for treatment to be effective. Therefore, there are campaigns to help prevent cervical cancer. The first is by the HPV vaccine which is given to girls of a secondary school age to prevent the spread of viruses (HPV-16 and HPV-18 strains) which are known to increase the risk of cervical cancer. The second is by cervical screening, where the cells of a woman's cervix are examined, once every few years, to look for changes to cell structure, as that can sometimes be an indication of cancer."

7. How does MRI work?

"MRI (magnetic resonance imaging) is a method of scanning the body using radio-waves and a large magnet, without the risk of radiation. An individual lies down a couch and is passed through the MRI scanner, which resembles a short tunnel. As the person passes through the scanner, the magnet creates a detailed picture of all the organs and bones using radio-waves and the magnetic field. This technique can identify pathology such as tumours on the images produced."

Patient.co.uk is an excellent resource to learn more about the types of medical investigations. It is definitely worth reading through some of the more commonly performed investigations such as ECG, X-ray, MRI, and Ultrasound.

8. How does Ultrasound imaging work?

"Ultrasound imaging is a painless way of viewing organs and structures inside the body using sound waves, which are transmitted through a hand held probe. Cold lubricating jelly is put on the area of skin to be scanned, and then the probe is held to the skin. Ultrasound waves are then sent through the probes. As the ultrasound waves hit the bones and organs, they bounce back towards the probe and a picture of all visible internal structures is formed."

9. What is the structure of DNA?

This question sounds simple but make sure your answer includes details about the structure of DNA and not about DNA in general. Try to explain the answer simply, without using lots of jargon as that could confuse you (unless you know the topic well).

"DNA is made up of a number of different molecules. The backbone is two strands of nucleotides, which run in opposite directions, and therefore are antiparallel. Nucleotides are made up of a base, a sugar group, and a phosphate group. There are four bases, adenine, thymine, guanine, and cytosine. As they all have unique structures, adenine is always joined to thymine on the opposite strand, and cytosine is always joined to *guanine. The strands are joined by ester bonds. The bases are assembled in a specific sequence, determining the genetic code."*

10. What is Down's syndrome?

"Down's syndrome is one of the most common types of genetic disease. It occurs when a person has three copies of chromosome 21 instead of two, usually due to a defect during cell replication in the production of the female egg. The greater the age of the mother, the higher the risk of her baby having Down's syndrome. This is particularly significant in women over the age of 40. The risk of Down's syndrome can be assessed during pregnancy, and if a mother is found to be at high risk, she

can be offered amniocentesis. This is a test which can determine if a baby has Down's syndrome by sampling the amniotic fluid but it does carry a risk of miscarriage. Down's syndrome is associated with a number of other medical conditions, the most common being problems with the structure of the heart."

11. **What are the differences between diseases in developing countries and those faced in the UK?**

This is testing knowledge of a subject known as epidemiology (study of the spread of diseases). To answer this question, think about what you may have heard on the news/read in the BMJ about the common health problems affecting both population groups, and what kind of diseases might these health problems cause.

"Many of the diseases in developing countries are due to poverty, inadequate diets and consumption of polluted water. These diseases include malnutrition (which although is not a disease in itself, it contributes to illnesses by weakening the immune system), gastroenteritis and other water-borne diseases. In the UK, diseases are often associated with involvement in activities that function as risk factors for these diseases. Risk factors such as smoking, drinking excessively, and obesity, are linked to a large proportion of diseases in this country including lung cancer, liver disease, and heart disease."

12. **Where are cholera and typhoid found and what are their symptoms?**

Make sure you answer the question being asked.

"Cholera and typhoid are both infections of the small intestine caused by ingesting bacteria, found in contaminated food or water. Both cholera and typhoid cause watery diarrhoea, of which typhoid may also cause blood in the stools, nausea and headaches. Cholera is usually found in parts of Africa, Asia, the Middle East and South America, whereas typhoid occurs mainly in the Indian subcontinent."

13. **What is the most common genetic disorder in the UK?**

"Genetic disorders usually vary according to race. Among Caucasians, the most common genetic disorder is cystic fibrosis which is due to a mutation in transmembrane conductance regulator, disrupting the transport of chloride and sodium ions across cell membranes. Among the African-Caribbean population the most common genetic disorder is sickle cell anaemia which is due to a mutation in the beta chain which makes haemoglobin in red blood cells."

14. **Can you describe how Down's syndrome manifests in a child?**

"Down's syndrome can vary in its severity. In most cases, a child may have some degree of learning disability. Furthermore, children with

Down's syndrome may have facial features as well as other physical characteristics, such as short stature. They may also suffer from problems with certain organs such as the heart and the intestines."

15. Which piece of imaging equipment do you consider to be the most important?

With this question there is no single right answer, but as always you should be able to justify your choice.

"I believe the X-ray machine to be the most important as although it is not as detailed as a CT scan or an MRI, it is usually by performing an X-ray that we identify that a problem is present, whereas CT and MRI mainly help confirm what

we have found on X-ray. "

16. Why are x-rays potentially dangerous?

X-rays are potentially dangerous as they cause radiation to pass through the body. If a high level of radiation passes through the body (due to lots of X-rays or CT scans being performed) this can cause the cells to undergo changes. This can cause damage to the cells, and can potentially contribute to cancer.

17. Describe the process of fertilisation.

"When a man and a woman have intercourse, sperm is propelled into a woman's vagina in a process known as ejaculation. The sperm then swim up through the vagina and cervix. If this occurs close to ovulation (day 14 of the

menstrual cycle), then an egg may be present in the womb. If so, one sperm forms a union with the egg. If this is successful and leads to the formation of a viable zygote - new life is created. "

18. Why is there no vaccination for the common cold?

"The common cold is caused by a number of different types of cold viruses (ranging from 200-700 types) and these are capable of mutating very quickly. Once a virus mutates, a vaccination against the virus is no longer effective and a constant supply of new vaccinations would be required to keep up with the rate of mutations. This is an unrealistic

prospect.

19. What problems are caused by obesity?

"Obesity contributes to a number of different health problems such as hypertension, diabetes, heart disease, osteoarthritis and stroke. It also causes a financial burden on the NHS for managing these diseases, as well as social problems such as discrimination, mobility issues, bullying in childhood obesity and segregation."

20. Name an antibiotic.

Examples include penicillin, amoxicillin, vancomycin, and gentamicin.

21. Why do we form scars from wounds?

"Scars are formed from wounds by the production of new collagen after injury to the skin. They close up the wound and prevent infection and further injury. "

22. What is a retrovirus?

"A retrovirus is a virus with a RNA genome surrounded by an envelope. It replicates making a DNA intermediate by reverse transcriptase."

23. Describe the transmission of an impulse across a synapse.

"When an action potential reaches the end of the pre-synaptic neurone, the voltage-gated calcium channels open causing calcium ions to flow into the cell. These ions cause synaptic vesicles to fuse with

the pre-synaptic membrane and empty their neurotransmitter chemicals into the synapse by exocytosis. These chemical diffuse across the synaptic cleft towards the post-synaptic neurone and bind to neuroreceptors on the membrane. This causes the channels to open and depolarization to occur, initiating an action potential, providing the threshold is reached. Certain enzymes are recruited to breakdown the excess neurotransmitter chemicals in the synapse and the products are reabsorbed by the pre-synaptic membrane by endocytosis. This stops activation of the post-synaptic neurone and therefore ceases to initiate action potentials. "

24. What is an ECG?

"ECG stands for electrocardiogram and it records a graphical representation of the heart's electrical activity and rhythm."

25. What is herd immunity?

"Herd immunity is a form of immunity when a population is vaccinated against a certain infectious disease which is spread by human contact. It makes it more difficult for that disease to be transmitted through the population and infect those who are not immunised."

26. Describe the problems with embryonic stem cells.

Stem cell biology is one of the most exciting areas of medicine and it may have a beneficial role in degenerative diseases such as diabetes, Parkinson's disease and heart failure. A stem cell is an undifferentiated cell that has to capacity to firstly self renew, and secondly to differentiate into more specialised cells in the body. For this question, most students discuss the ethical, political and legal issues surrounding embryonic stem cells, however for bonus points, it is important to include the biological difficulties to overcome in your answer.

"There are a number of different problems with embryonic stem cells in each of the fields of ethics, law and biology. Ethical issues include, questioning the moral status of the embryo and comparisons have been between use of embryos and killing babies. This is completely untrue since stem cells come from the embryo at the blastocyst stage and they are just a few

cells. *Other accusations include ideas that stem cell research is playing God, however, one could argue that this is something that doctors always do e.g. prescribing aspirin to prevent a future stroke and the Hippocratic oath necessitates us to act like this. In UK the government is relatively supportive of stem cell research, however on the other side of the Atlantic, this is not the case. Therefore, in the UK we are lucky that stem cell research is permitted as it can have a beneficial outcome on how we treat diseases in the future.* Lastly, the biological issues with stem cells are firstly that they are capable of causing an immune response since the cells are non-host, unlike adult cells, and secondly that they are tumourgenic and are therefore prone to developing into unstable tumours."

Chapter 3

<u>Ethical Based Questions</u>

When answering ethical questions, there is usually no single right answer, but certain themes/points of view may need to be presented. When asked questions where an opinion is needed, try to present a balanced argument, even if you have a strong opinion on the matter, to show you have weighed up and considered all the options.

It is important that you are aware of the Hippocratic Oath, the 4 principles of medical ethics and its importance in the clinical setting.

1. **If you were given £100,000 to spend on a developing country, how would you use it?**

   With this question, try to think of sensible (not necessarily medical) ways of spending money which would address issues in the developing world. For example donating money towards:

   - *"Water sanitation to ensure constant clean water supply as gastroenteritis is the most common cause of death in children less than age 5 in the developing world.*
   - *The buying and growing of crops and farm equipment in rural areas to form a sustainable food supply/provision of long lasting goods. Make sure you raise the point about the*

possibility of goods falling into the wrong hands and ending up on the black market.

- *Academic resources such as exercise books, textbooks and writing tools can be used as resources for poor schools."*

It is also important to think of contributing to projects that are sustainable and will have a long lasting impact on the community.

2. **Is death acceptable for a Jehovah witness if they refuse blood transfusions?**

With ethical questions there is very rarely one correct answer, a balanced argument is more important.

N.B. Jehovah's witnesses can accept blood components, just not whole blood.

"Due to patient autonomy a patient has the right to refuse treatment as long as their doctor has explained the consequences of not having the treatment, including death. However, despite patient choice, each patient also has the right to be treated. Therefore, if an alternative was possible such as giving blood components, then this should be performed instead."

3. **If, on a scale of 0 to 5, 0 was caring for people and 5 was an interest in science, where would you put yourself on the scale?**

As medicine combines the art of caring for people as well as an interest in science, it wouldn't be advisable to select either 0 or 5 as that would imply you lack one of the core attributes of being a doctor. If you place yourself towards either end of the scale make sure you acknowledge the other quality as being important in medicine.

"As I have a strong interest in both caring for people and an interest in science, I would put myself as a 3, especially as I feel both of these attributes are essential for a doctor to have."

4. **Would you feel emotionally affected if a patient died?**

A question like this is trying to ascertain whether you appreciate the range of emotions you will feel due to the situations you experience during your time in medicine. It would also be important to highlight the emotional strength that is required to be a good doctor.

"Being human, I think I would feel emotional if a patient died, such as sadness for the patient and their family, anger that despite our best efforts a patient still died, or even relief that the patient's suffering had ended. However, I know that in medicine there will be many scenarios which will challenge me emotionally, and it is important to find a healthy way to deal with these instances."

5. Why do you consider the suicide rate in doctors is high?

"Doctors can undergo severe mental stress due to the events they experience during their working life,

such as seeing patients of all ages die and having to juggle a pressurised job and working unsocial hours, combined with having a family. Often doctors feel they cannot talk to others about their problems, as it was previously seen as a sign of weakness to show that one needed help. One could argue that this lead to doctors 62nternalizing their problems. Unfortunately, in quite a number of cases, the problems experienced are serious enough that doctors feel they cannot cope and feel there is no way out other than suicide. Furthermore, doctors often have access to potentially harmful medications and as such any attempted suicide is more likely to be successful with their medical knowledge and resources."

6. **What do you think of stem cell research and the possibility of using it to treat diabetes?**

    "Stem cell research has been an exciting area of medicine over the last decade, as there is the potential that stem cells could be used to regenerate organs. Although progress has been made, it may take years before stem cell research is widely used to cure what are known as autoimmune diseases (diseases where the body does not recognise a particular organ as being a part of itself and it begins to attack itself), e.g. diabetes (where the pancreas is affected) and thyroid disease. In diabetes, it is thought that stem cell research could be used to 'grow' another pancreas using the patient's own stem cells, and see whether this would stop

the body attacking it."

7. Would you empathise or sympathise?

The definition of empathy is the ability to identify with another person's feelings and emotionally put oneself in the place of another. Sympathy is feeling pity or sorrow for the misfortune of others.

"Even though sympathy is our normal reaction to hearing someone's bad news, I would empathise more than sympathise as I think it is more important for a patient to know that their doctor understands what they are going through, even without going through it themselves, compared to a doctor who just feels sorry for them."

8. **Would you think that you have failed if one of your patients die?**

Interviewers are once again looking for the human element to your work. Try to be honest; acknowledging that you may feel like a failure, but show that you understand that a doctor cannot carry those feelings around as it may affect their work.

"Death is something that doctors face on a daily basis and of course it would be difficult to accept the death of one of my own patients. However, after analysing my own actions to ensure that there was nothing more I could have done and having worked to the best of my ability to save this patient, I would not let

myself feel that I have failed."

9. **Do you know the four ethical principles of medicine?**

1. *"Respect for **Autonomy** - the patient has the right to refuse or choose their treatment.*

2. *Principle of **Beneficence** - a practitioner should always act in the best interest of the patient.*

3. *Principle of **Non-maleficence** – a practitioner should never do harm to a patient.*

4. *Principle of **Justice** – this is about the distribution of scarce health resources and the decision of who gets what treatment."*

10. **Do you believe an alcoholic has the same rights as a non-alcoholic to receive treatment and potentially a transplant?**

Main point with this question is not to be judgmental.

"As one of the foundations of medicine is that everyone has the right to receive treatment without prejudice, regardless of their lifestyle, I believe alcoholics have the right to receive treatment. However, as a prerequisite for receiving a transplant is evidence that the patient will look after the transplanted organ, in the same way a smoker would be required to give up smoking before receiving a transplant, an alcoholic may not be eligible to undergo a

liver transplant unless they show evidence that they have stopped drinking. As long as the patient has stopped drinking for the required amount of time, the patient is entitled to receive a transplant in the same way as any other patient."

11. Do you believe euthanasia is acceptable? Explain why.

As said previously, it is important in these types of questions to present both sides of the argument.

"I believe in cases where a patient has a disabling illness which worsens their quality of life, and where the chances of recovery are slim to none, I believe euthanasia may be acceptable

only if suggested by the patient themselves. As doctors are primarily promoters of health I do not think it is appropriate for doctors to ever suggest it. However, I do not think euthanasia is an acceptable option for every person suffering from a chronic illness, as many people with chronic illnesses are still able to maintain a good quality of life."

12. **Do you think those who have physical disabilities should be allowed to practice medicine?**

"If an individual's disability does not reduce their capacity to learn what is required to practice medicine, care for their patients and impart knowledge to others, then yes I feel *individuals with physical disabilities should be allowed to practice medicine. However, it does need to be acknowledged that these individuals may have extra needs which would need to be addressed."*

13. Is it fair for the NHS to dedicate time and resources to patients who have self-inflicted conditions?

With this question, regardless of personal opinion you have to show that you know the NHS was created to treat everyone, regardless of whether an individual is to blame for their conditions.

23. *"As the NHS was created to treat everyone, even if their condition is self-inflicted, our job is*

simply to treat these individuals. Still, in this current economic climate and the financial problems the NHS are facing, we cannot ignore the time and resources lost treating these individuals, which could have been used on other patients. Rather than lay blame on these patients, I think it is more important to take preventative steps which would reduce the number of individuals with self-inflicted diseases, promoting healthy lifestyles such as reducing alcohol intake, stopping smoking and encouraging a healthy diet and exercise regime."

14. **Would you operate on an obese person despite knowing that the operation's effects**

may be void in 6 months for example with a hip replacement?

Here is an opportunity to show that you know the ethical pillars of medicine (look at the question on ethical pillars of medicine if you do not know what they are), and to show that you understand that quality of life is extremely important in making such decisions.

*"I would do the operation as it would improve the quality of life for that patient. However, I would ensure they were aware that if they did not lose weight they would go back to the way they were. If the patient still wanted the operation, as the first ethical ***pillar*** of medicine is respect for autonomy I would*

perform the surgery."

15. Is it okay for doctors to experience personal feelings towards their patients?

I do not think they are interpreting personal feelings as romantic feelings, so unless you want to find yourself pulled up in front of the GMC before you even become a doctor do not say you think romantic feelings are allowed!

"As doctors are the first and foremost people, it is normal that some patients may evoke feelings of frustration, joy, sadness or even anger. However, it is important that doctors are able to prevent these feelings from clouding their judgment both positively (being more attentive to one patient at the detriment of the other)

and negatively."

16. Do you think doctors should have the right to strike?

A doctor's first responsibility is toward their patients, however, as doctors have to make a living too, if they decided they needed to take a stand against something, I believe doctors are allowed to strike providing they ensure patient care is not compromised.

Recently doctors took strike action in order to prevent changes to pensions which would involve larger contributions for a smaller pension and 2 extra years of service. Supported by the BMA, the strike action meant that those who participated cancelled all non-essential procedures and clinics, whilst emergency services ran as normal. This caused major disruption but wasn't considered to have been a cause of human death. Again, as with any opinion based question, weigh up the arguments to sound well rounded.

"I think that doctors should be allowed to strike as any other profession is, as they should be allowed to express their discontent about the things which concern their livelihood. The recent strike action which took place concerning pensions, highlighted that strike action can cause maximal disruption while not jeopardising human life too much. Although I do understand why it is thought that doctors should not be

allowed to strike as the nature of their job means looking after vulnerable individuals who without their care could die. Additionally, having happier, more in control doctors also means having a happier more efficient healthcare team."

17. What are the arguments for and against a ban on selling tobacco?

This is to see whether you are able to think laterally about a controversial topic. It is important to look at both sides of the question as it specifically says "for and against".

"With the occurrence of lung cancer on the rise, Tobacco selling is still a controversial issue. Tobacco selling should be banned as it leads to

an increase in the number of young people who take up smoking. However, as all individuals have the right to choose whether to smoke or not, putting a blanket ban on the sale of tobacco may lead to the recurring argument that Britain is turning into a nanny state."

18. **What is more important; quality of life or length of life?**

Quality of life is an important factor in medicine in determining the impact of disease, medication, or any intervention on a person's life. It is usually regarded as more important than the length of a person's life within medicine.

"Although we would all like to live long lives,

above all I believe it's more important to live a fulfilled life, no matter its length. Therefore, I think quality of life is more important than length of life."

19. What are the arguments for and against abortion?

There is no right or wrong answer to this question but it is important to give both sides of the argument with the support of evidence. As a medical student and future doctor, you will have to reach your own decision on where you stand with the ethics of abortion and therefore, the interviewers want to see if you are well-informed on this controversial topic. The law states that a fetus is not a person until it is born and that it does not have rights. For abortion to be granted and pregnancy not to take place, the pregnancy must be terminated by a registered practitioner, providing two registered practitioners are of the same opinion formed. It is important that you know details about the abortion law, as you may be asked this in your interview and it is worth looking it up.

"There are a number of arguments for and against abortion. Arguments for abortion are; the fetus has no rights, parents do not have a duty to protect their children, in cases of rape, the woman has not consented for another human being to occupy her uterus, the mother has a right to decide what should happen to her body, abortion is seen as a failure to rescue as opposed to active killing and lastly if the fetus has a serious disease, it will impact on the care it will receive from the mother and therefore abortion should be allowed. Arguments against abortions are based on the reasoning that the fetus has rights; the fetus is a person from day 14 or conception, the fetus has the potential to become a person and has as much right to live as a child who has been born."

20. Why is it important to learn about ethics?

"Medical ethics helps to shed light on the moral situations which medical students and future doctors unavoidably face on a daily basis. Ethical awareness is a vital part of becoming a good doctor and learning the principles or pillars of medical ethics can assist in making difficult decisions."

21. What are the advantages and disadvantages of a private health care system?

As with other questions, make sure you provide a balanced argument and structure your answer logically.

"The advantages of privatisation include a better outcome for treatment, more personalised care, more efficient and effective care, and reduced waiting times and faster referrals. The disadvantages of privatisation are that the profit goes to the shareholders, money is wasted as unnecessary investigations are carried out, and medical care would no longer be a public service."

22. Should the HPV vaccine be available on the NHS?

"There are two vaccines called Garasil and Cervarix, also known as the 'HPV vaccine' which is given to girls aged 12-13 to prevent the development of cervical cancer (2nd most common cancer in women under age 35) and genital warts in young females. The human papilloma virus (HPV) spreads through skin to skin sexual contact and it can only be treated, not cured. There has been some disagreement as to whether having this vaccine available on the NHS was appropriate, even though it is potentially life-saving. Administration of the HPV vaccine is believed to send out an inappropriate message, as it approves of sexual activity at a young age. In fact, there are also arguments that girls become more promiscuous in believing that are safe from HPV infections, although the vaccine only protects against 4 types of the virus.

This could increase teen pregnancies as well as the incidence of sexually transmitted diseases. Other groups such as those associated with religion also objected to the vaccine being available on the NHS as they felt it was not applicable to girls who are not sexually active and remaining celibate until marriage. However, these individuals may still be exposed to different forms of the HPV and this vaccine protects against them. Although society is changing, it is unlike that girls aged 12 or 13 understand the full purpose of the vaccine and it is therefore unlikely to increase teen pregnancies. Condoms can be used for protection against HPV, however it can still spread very easily from one person to another and so this vaccine is vital and should remain on the NHS childhood vaccination programme."

Why did you choose to apply for Medicine at this particular university?

1. Tell me about yourself and something interesting you have done?

Never lie in this type of question! Not everyone will have had the opportunity to go trekking in the Himalayas or assist in surgery before they get to medical school, and if you say you have done something you haven't and are asked about it in your interview, it could be a disaster. Think about what makes you different from everybody else...this may be a particular talent or the way you have used a gift. If you have difficulty thinking of something interesting about yourself ask those who know you best such as family and friends to describe you in a few words. Also try not to make this sound like an advert for a dating website.

"I am generally an outgoing person, and enjoy both sporting (mainly netball) and creative hobbies, such as singing and playing the piano. I enjoy working with children and have done so over many years through various summer jobs as a nursery assistant. Through my involvement with my church choir I was selected to captain a choir course held by the Royal School of Church Music. This role involved being responsible for 30 girls where I was able to develop my

leadership and communication skills."

2. What can you contribute to this university?

This is a good place to mention your extracurricular activities such as sports you play/clubs you are involved in at school which you would like to continue at university. If you have played to regional/national levels it is a good idea to mention it. Also mention activities such as fundraising, expeditions, dance/drama performances you have participated in. This is because as well as the most academically able students, universities look for students who are able to contribute to university in other ways.

"Having been a keen netballer for most of my school days, and being part of a team that has

won both regional and national tournaments, I would be keen to continue playing netball at '(insert name of university)'. Furthermore, during my time as House Captain in sixth form I co-ordinated our entry for the inter-house music competition and our entry for the inter-house drama competition, for which we came first and second respectively. I discovered I really enjoyed both performing in, and planning productions so would enjoy the opportunity to do this at university."

3. **What do you know about the way we teach medicine?**

Research the course at each university you are applying to as there are significant differences between them. Know whether your course is traditional (i.e. 2 years of lecture based medical sciences followed by 3 years of clinical sciences), integrated (where you learn clinical science alongside medical science), problem based learning (where teaching is based around a problem presented which often includes a lot of self study) and whether the course includes dissection of cadavers, or whether simulated dissection takes place.

"At Kings, the medical course is taught quite traditionally. During the first two years teaching is very lecture based, mainly focusing on the medical sciences such as anatomy, biochemistry and physiology, as well as including basic clinical skills such as how to examine the

cardiovascular and respiratory system. During the 'clinical' years teaching is less structured, and more learning is to be gleaned on the wards. However, occasional lectures still occur."

4. **What are the different type of medical degree programmes?**

Different universities offer different courses, so become familiar with the courses that run at your prospective universities so you are able to talk about them.

"Generally speaking, the most common program is the five year program. This is run at most medical schools in the country, and accepts both school leavers and graduates. Some universities, such as Bart's and GKT offer *an accelerated four year degree programme for post graduate students. Other universities (including GKT) offer an extended medical degree, providing extra assistance to those from disadvantaged schools/areas. Other courses include the foundation course, which in essence is a pre-medical year, providing grounding in the sciences and maths for those missing all or an element of these subjects."*

5. What do you know about intercalated BSc?

"The intercalated BSc is a one year degree programme which can be obtained alongside your medical degree. It is usually taken after the second year of medicine, but can also be taken after third and fourth year. Although this

degree is usually in a medically related subject, such as Pharmacology or Physiology, there is wide variety of programmes available, which vary by university. The intercalated BSc provides a student with the opportunity to study an area of interest in detail, with the potential to undertake research and have that research published."

6. If you like the systems based course, why did you apply to Cambridge?

Even though this particular question is related to Cambridge University, it highlights the importance of knowing the differences between medical courses offered at various universities, in particular knowing the courses at the universities you have applied to. This information can be found via University websites, and is usually found under 'course outline'.

"Although Cambridge does not have a systems based course, I like the fact that students are taught the theory of medicine (medical sciences), enabling them to apply this knowledge to the practice of medicine."

7. **Explain your choices of university on your UCAS form.**

It is important to that you show you have done your research on your chosen universities.

"Main reasons can include: location (if close to home, you can commute), course type, interest

in research performed (look on university website to see what research is being performed), entry requirements."

8. **What extra-curricular activities would you consider joining here if you were offered a place?**

This question is a chance to 'show off' your previous sporting or artistic achievements, or to show an aspect of your personality by talking about different activities you would like to be a part of. Ones such as MSF and Red Cross can show your awareness of medical campaign groups. You can go onto the University's student union website to have a look at what clubs and societies are held, and decide which activities you would be interested in. If you choose a slightly unusual group/society be prepared to discuss why.

"Having played netball to a high standard at my school, I would relish the opportunity to represent my university in this way. Furthermore, I would also be interested in joining the volunteer groups YELP and SHINE; which both involve working with children from surrounding areas and deprived schools. I was involved in mentoring younger students at school, and found it humbling to see the positive impact on the children involved."

9. **What are you going to do for us, without mentioning your academic achievements?**

Similarly to the question above, this is an opportunity to talk about your previous non-academic achievements in the context of activities you would like to continue, or you can go onto the University's student union website and decide which activities appeal to you.

"Being a keen singer, I would like to continue this by joining the university choir. Having played netball to a high standard at my school, I would relish the opportunity to represent my university in this way. Furthermore, as I have been involved in charity work during school, I would like to continue this in some form at university. I am also interested in volunteering abroad and combining this with charity work in groups such as Tenteleni or the Kenyan Orphan

Project."

10. **You said you like the course structure here, how do you think the Systems and Topics based structure here is going to help the future of Medicine?**

"It will help the future of medicine because it is a method of ensuring that all the necessary facts are taught in a way that students will find easier to digest. It allows compartmentalization of the vast information needed to be learnt, increasing the likelihood that the facts will be remembered."

It is important to do some research about the structure of the programmes at the individual institution, these are constantly changing so it is always a good idea to look at an up-to-date prospectus.

11. What are the qualities about our medical school that attract you the least?

When asked to comment on a negative aspect of your course or university, always include an explanation of how you could overcome it. This will show the interviewer that you can take initiative and be resourceful.

"As Kings College London School of Medicine is the largest medical school in Europe; the least attractive quality may be the size of the cohort. If I was lucky enough to gain a place at this medical school if I would ensure I knew who to contact if I required academic or personal

support."

12. What do you know about PBL? Why do you want to come to a PBL medical school?

PBL (problem based learning) is something all prospective medical students need to be aware of, even more so if you are applying to a University that teaches by PBL, such as Bart's.

"PBL, or problem based learning is a relatively new way of facilitating learning amongst medical students. Opposed to the more traditional way of teaching (known as didactic) by lectures, PBL presents students with a 'problem' in a tutorial, and with the help of a facilitator, address the issues raised in the problem. I would like to go to a PBL medical

school as I feel I learn better by being more actively involved in my education, by being able to have discussions with peers, as opposed to being sat in a lecture room with 100 other students."

Chapter 5

Personal qualities about you based questions

1. What makes you a good doctor?

To answer this question, you need to know
what qualities are necessary for a doctor to
have. Most medical schools have a list of
qualities they expect doctors, and therefore
medical students to have. This can usually be
found on their school of medicine website or in
the prospectus so it is worth having a look
through that list. When answering personality-
based questions such as this, rather than just
listing qualities, pick two or three and provide

evidence that you possess these skills.

"First and foremost I believe I would be a good doctor because I have a strong interest in both science and people. I have had an interest in science early on at school, and it was this interest that lead to me studying Chemistry and Biology at A level. During Human Biology lessons I found I always wanted to know the reason why things went wrong in the body during disease, and it was this questioning that really fired my interest in the human body. Since I have been old enough to have a job, I have always had a job which involved lots of interaction with the public, especially children. Through both paid and volunteer work I have worked with people of all ages, through my *work at a Care home, a nursery nurse assistant,*

a math's and science tutor, as a waitress and a

retail assistant. The aspect I always enjoyed the

most was talking to people. I feel my passion for

people and for science, twinned with my good

communication skills, provide a excellent

foundation, which if built upon appropriately

would make me a good doctor."

2. Take us through your personal statement?

As everyone's personal statement is different it

is impossible to come up with a model answer

for this question, but this question highlights

that you need to know your personal statement

well. You should also be able to draw attention

to what you regard as the highlights of your

statement. This should include all the points that make you stand out from the crowd, as well as your academic ability and anything else that you feel shows your competence as a prospective medical student.

3. **How did you prepare for this interview?**

To prepare for this interview I read over my personal statement, ensuring I knew everything I mentioned. For the last few weeks I have also been reading the New Scientist to keep up with recent scientific advances. I have also had a look at the university website over the last couple of weeks to see whether any new research has been published.

4. **What qualities make a poor doctor?**

Begin by saying how although individuality among doctors is encouraged, there are certain qualities which would not be helpful within the medical field. Such qualities include:

- Poor timekeeping

- Inability to work in a team

- Poor communication skills

- Poor record keeping

5. **How has your journey been thus far?**

"As with most journeys, my education has been generally smooth. Some parts have been very rewarding, such as winning academic prizes during my time in school and sixth form, and other parts have been somewhat more

challenging, but I have managed to overcome them. I know that if given the opportunity to begin a degree in medicine, that there will be greater academic challenges ahead, but I am confident that I will find methods to overcome them."

6. Do you eat healthily?

"I generally do. I try to eat a balanced diet with lots of fruit and vegetables, as well as keeping an eye on my portion size. However, these good habits tend to go out of the window during revision!"

7. Do you have any family in the medical profession, if so have they influenced you in any way to become a doctor?

The following model question is for people who have medical professionals in the family. However, if you have no family in the medical profession you can discuss how a family member's encounter with doctors influenced your decision to be a doctor.

"My aunt is a doctor, and hearing the passion she had for her job, made me want to find out more about the profession. Furthermore, on doing some work experience with her at her GP practice, I admired the way she interacted with patients and always tried to do her best for them. It showed me how important good communication skills are in medicine, as they can determine whether or not a patient follows your advice. Due to her influence I have tried to

improve my communication skills as well as

maintain a good level of academic

achievement."

8. What do you do to relax?

This question is just to show the panel that you

know how to relax, and have a life outside of

medicine. It does not need to be anything

exciting.

"I like to relax at home with family and friends

watching films or just talking. I also like to play

netball and play the piano to relax."

9. Sell yourself to us for 2 minutes?

With questions such as these it is important

that you say things about yourself that you can

back up if possible, e.g. by talking about achievements, prizes, anything that makes you stand out.

"Not only am I academically able but I am excelling in my studies as shown by the prize I won at school for academic excellence and all round achievement. I also have a wide range of interests. I have played netball for my school, including representing the school at the National Independent Schools Tournament, winning both a gold and silver medal in the competition. I am also quite musical, having played the piano for a number of years, and achieving a grade 5 in piano. I also sing in my church, and have sung with the Royal School of Church Music on a number of occasions. I love

working with children, and have done so over the last 2 summers as a nursery nurse assistant."

10. Do you read? What was the last book you read?

This question is just to ensure that you have outside interests.

"I love to read, the last book I read was called 'Handle with Care' by Jodi Picoult. This is about a child born with severe osteogenesis imperfecta whose mother takes the decision to sue the doctor who delivered her child for wrongful birth. The book details how each member of her family handled the illness, and the impact of the trial on each on them."

11. What genre of films or books are you most interested in?

This question is just to ensure that you have outside interests.

"I enjoy a wide variety of books and films, but mostly drama, comedy and romance."

For questions 62 and 63 the panel usually want to assess your ability to communicate in a professional manner, avoid jargon and give an honest answer.

12. Are you a people person or do you prefer to be alone?

"Generally I am a people person, and enjoy activities like going out for meals with friends,

but I enjoy being in my own company occasionally."

13. Do you enjoy working in a team?

"I enjoy working in a team, and have worked in many different teams such as sports teams, the charity committee at school, where we raised money throughout the year for a charity of our choice, and through my work as a House Captain, which included putting on our own production."

14. Have you ever experienced death?

In answering a question like this the interview panel want to see your human side, and the thoughts we have surrounding death. Even though in medicine we are required to separate our emotions from our job, that's not to say we should not experience emotion at all.

"I have experienced death in different ways. Firstly when I was 14, my cousin died after being diagnosed with a brain tumour. As she had been an inpatient in hospital for a number of weeks, her death almost provided relief. Secondly, on my first day shadowing a doctor at a hospital, a patient went into cardiac arrest and died in front of me. This was an interesting way to see death as it was at such close proximity, however, as I had neither seen nor interacted with the patient, I felt slightly detached from the situation. Thirdly my grandfather passed away a few months ago, and this was the most difficult of all the deaths I

have experienced to cope with. All three experiences were very different, but they have all made me appreciate life in a new way."

15. Medicine is a very long and stressful subject to study, how do you deal with stress?

"I have a very strong support network of both friends and family who help me in times of stress by enabling me to talk about any problems I may be having. I have also found that exercise, and going for walks help me deal with stress."

16. Tell me about any of the situations where you have shown leadership skills.

"I used teamwork as well as leadership skills in my role as a House Captain, where I was

responsible for producing and directing a theatre production. I had to audition students for roles, and allocate other students for backstage roles. I would then oversee rehearsals, and liaise with the students responsible for costumes, music and stage props. As I was dealing with 15 girls between the ages of 11 and 17 I had to assert my authority at times. Thankfully the production was a success!"

17. **In ten years time after you have become a doctor and all your friends want to have a reunion but you are unable to attend, how would you want them to remember you?**

"I would want them to remember me as a girl

who got involved in all aspects of university life, who worked hard and played hard at appropriate times, and who made a significant contribution to some aspect of university life."

18. **What are the most important attributes for maintaining good working relationship between colleagues?**

Good working relationships are important to improve the communication flow, develop understanding of each other's views, reduce tensions and disagreements, and improve efficiency within any working environment. This is even more important in the multidisciplinary team approach undertaken in medicine today.

"Good communication is essential to any team

environment, to make sure everyone knows

what's going on, and that the team are all

working towards the same goal."

19. Do you do anything that involves working in a team?

"I have played in a netball team, representing my school at a National Tournament, and also sing in my church choir. I was also a House Captain, which involved working with the other prefects in the school. "

This can be any sport or group work that you are actively involved in.

20. How can you relate being a doctor to playing competitive sport?

"I think every doctor wants to be the top of their field, however, as in competitive sport this cannot be achieved alone. You need to be able to work with other members of your team, in this case, other healthcare professionals to become the best you can be. If you didn't do this in sport, you run the risk of losing the game; the equivalent of this in medicine would be causing a problem, even death in a patient."

21. Have you ever considered taking a gap year?

"I considered it very briefly, but as I was keen to start university I decided I would rather travel after completing my education.

However, if you have taken a gap year that can be advantageous especially if you participated in some form of health care or volunteering. If so, highlight in detail the nature of the work you did and how you feel it has made you a better medical candidate this time round."

22. Give examples of where you have used teamwork and leadership skills?

"I used teamwork and leadership skills in my role as a House Captain, where I was responsible for producing and directing a theatre production. I had to audition people for roles, and allocate other people backstage roles. I would then oversee rehearsals, and liaise with the people responsible for costumes, music and stage props. As I was dealing with 15 girls between the ages of 11 and 17 I had to assert

my authority at times. Thankfully the production was a success!"

23. What did you do for Duke of Edinburgh?

Try to highlight the points that display qualities that would be advantageous in medicine, such as resilience, and ability to work in a team.

"For my Duke of Edinburgh, I travelled to Ecuador with a group of other students. While we were there we helped build a school, as well as 'buddying' up with an Ecuadorian person around the same age as ourselves, to help them improve their English. As the building project was led by us we had to work together to build it successfully. Furthermore we trekked through the Amazon, where teamwork was essential for

us to avoid injury. This trek included scaling

mountains, a difficult task for most but nearly

impossible if one is afraid of heights like me.

However, due to resilience (and a lot of

encouragement from my peers) I was able to

reach the summit."

24. Have you ever had to make an unpopular decision as a leader?

Firstly explain your leadership role, and then detail the unpopular decision you made. If possible, think of an unpopular decision that had gained you the respect of your peers and also turned out to be the correct decision for the situation.

"In my role as Deputy House Captain, we would

hold events such as inter-house music competition. Usually the final piece would be performed by one of the most talented musicians in the school, however, I decided to break with tradition and perform a group number. This was unpopular with not only other pupils performing in the show, but also the House Captain. This lead to a tense atmosphere in the lead up to the competition, but my decision was proven correct when we won the competition and received a special commendation for our group performance."

25. **Do you believe your communication and organisational skills are adequate to become a great doctor?**

Never say yes, as these can always be improved upon. This shows that you understand the need for continuous personal development.

"Although I feel I have very good communication and organisational skills, shown by previous roles I have held successfully such as House Captain while in Year 13, as well as participating heavily in church activities all the while without letting my academic standards slip; I feel that there is always more I can learn, and I hope that through experiences I hope to gain at medical school, my communication and organisation skills will develop further, therefore enabling me to eventually become a great doctor."

26. What do you do in your spare time?

Again the interviewing panel are looking for someone with outside interests. As said previously if you have a particularly interesting hobby then mention it, but otherwise just make whatever you do sound interesting.

27. What would you describe as your worst qualities?

I would advise against putting anything down which would cause interview panels to look at you less favourably, such as being a pathological liar. With whatever bad quality you name, try and show how it could be an advantage within medicine, but what you could do to try and master it.

Examples:

- Too nice: allow people to take me for granted

"One of my worst qualities is being too nice to everyone, as this allows people to take me for granted. However, I think that being too nice can certainly help you on the win over some of the more challenging patients. However, to improve this quality, I have tried to become more assertive, more vocal and less flexible when deemed necessary."

28. How would your closest friends describe you?

In this answer, try to give a range of positives which would give the questioner a wider insight into your personality that you may not have showed already. Sound genuine and use specific, descriptive words with examples of why your friends would describe you in that way.

"My closest friends would describe me as generous, as I am always willing to share what I have with them; as loyal as I will always be willing to stand with them in whatever they need help in doing and finally organised, as I seem to be the one who always has to organise the nights out!"

29. How do you handle criticism?

No one likes criticism but it is a necessary part of life in order to improve and grow as a person. It would be easy to say "I love criticism!" however, honesty in these situations shows that you can truly reflect on your own character flaws (if you do have them). Think about why you dislike criticism (if you actually do like it – please ignore) and use it to construct your answer.

"As a proud person, I am sensitive to the criticism that I receive. Howeve,r I believe that feedback, positive or negative, is an integral part of improving myself. When I receive criticism, I attempt to understand why it is being said and furthermore question the source about ways I can improve that aspect of myself."

At this point it would also be appropriate to insert a real life experience, giving an example of when you have had to deal with critique.

30. **Give me an example when you have had your opinions overridden, what did you do?**

In scenario questions, there will always be situations that you may or may not have encountered. The most important thing is that you think about the outcomes which would best reflect your character. If you are a strong willed person answer honestly, however, there is a fine line between trying to make your point heard and being argumentative. Come up with the most logical response so that it seems you are at least diplomatic in your thinking. However, do not compromise your personality completely by being a 'push-over'.

"While in a committee meeting.......my point about changing X.... was disregarded by members of the committee, particularly the chair person, and although I tried to clarify my point, I believe that when opposition for your idea comes from multiple sources, it is important to re-evaluate whether your opinion is as valid as you think it was. Hence, I took away the reasoning for the disagreement and came back in the next meeting with evidence for why I suggested such an action."

31. What is your ten year plan?

When planning your life start by outlining the initial dream, and then setting out the clear objectives which need to be achieved in order for this dream to come true. Goals and objectives must be SMART: **S**pecific, **M**easureable, **A**ttainable, **R**elevant, and **T**imely. In this vein, attempt to set yourself clear targets which you can reach within those ten years, possibly giving time frames of how long an objective will take to accomplish, hopefully born from some sort of research. Furthermore, they should have a clear measurable outcome which you can record as a success if you achieve them.

"Within ten years I hope to be a surgical trainee in Plastic Surgery and own two houses. In order to do this I would need to:

- *Have completed medical school*

- *Got a London deanery foundation job, hopefully in North East London.*

- *Be working on my portfolio with a range of activities, including publications, audits and teaching*

- *Passed my MRCS part A and B within my FY1-2 years*

- *Obtain a CT1 post within 4 years of graduating*

- *Obtain a ST3 post within 6 years of graduating*

- *Save £20K within 3 years of graduation to put down a deposit on my first property*

- *Use the capital from my first property within 6 years of owning to put down a deposit for the 2nd property, and rent out first."*

32. What person(s) has had the biggest positive impact on you?

This can be a personal question, however, it is a good opportunity to appreciate someone who has either inspired you through their words or actions as a role model, or someone who has directly contributed to your schooling or extra-curricular activities. Highlight the things you have learnt from them or how they have had an impact on your life. Finally, talk about how you have taken it on board or how this impact will develop you as a person.

"My coach at my football club, Ridgeway Rovers FC has been one of the most influential people in my life so far. Over the last 2 years playing

under his guidance, he has not only help me improved me as a footballer, but also instilled in me some of what he describes as the key values to succeeding in life. This includes hard work and dedication to your craft, making sure you are early to the things you need to be on time to, and finally having the confidence in yourself succeed in the task ahead of you. These are some of the things which I have tried to apply not only to my sporting life, but more importantly to my personal and academic life and have helped me through much of my A levels so far."

33. How have you developed your communication skills?

The only way to develop your communication skills is to use your communication skills. Hence, before you can answer a question like this, you should have already been taking part in activities which will actually develop the skill of talking and listening effectively to people. Activities such as taking part in debates, presentations, talks and public speaking help in showing that you have been able to display your communication skills. Meanwhile actively taking part in workshops, teaching sessions, and activity groups which focus on improving communications show that you have a keenness to improve. However, remember that almost every aspect of human life today requires good communication to be successful, so highlighting activities which shows your personal progression or improvement in your communication skills could be a more tactful way to answer a question like this.

The interviewer(s) will immediately know from the first time you answer a question whether you have good communication skills, and so this is much more than a tick box exercise. Medicine is about communication and so you should think about developing your communication skills constantly to help you become a good medical student and future doctor. Skills are the tools you have to carve out your future. Therefore, like any useful tool it needs to sharpened and ready to be used as any moment...

Chapter 6

Work experience and education based questions

1. How are your A-levels going?

Not great? Is it a case of how would you LIKE your A-levels to be going? If they are going as well as you have hoped so far, say so and give the reasons why. However, if they haven't been as straightforward as they could have been, make sure you sound positive or at the very least optimistic! Again, like with any question, giving examples is imperative.

"This year doing my A-levels has been the most challenging time of my school life to date, with more independence over my learning while taking in new ideas and ways of thinking through the questions put to us, particularly in my science subjects. However, it has also been enjoyable as I have been able to see myself grow as a person and become more responsible for my own learning and understanding. It has driven me to continue to work hard at the topics which I am weakest at."

2. **How would any non-science subject at GCSE/A-level help as a doctor?**

Being a good doctor requires more than just scientific knowledge. As a doctor, you will play many roles; the communicator, the mediator, the presenter, the investigator. Therefore, it is essential for any doctor to be versatile both in their skills and way of thinking. That is why doing non-science subject at GSCE and A levels can be a great benefit in developing more than just your scientific skills. Subjects like History, Law and Criminology help to critically analyse sources, while Psychology and Sociology help us understand human behaviours. They can all play a part in shaping you as a doctor so don't be afraid to admit your interest in the different subjects that you have taken as long as you can justify how it can help mould you into the best possible doctor you can be.

"As a doctor, I believe you need to be a well-rounded and conscientious individual in order to have perspective on some of the major clinical decisions which you will be taking, which can have huge implications on the lives of the patients who you treat. Hence, I believe that having knowledge and experience of alternative subjects which broaden the way that you interpret and understand the world beneficial. Having studied Psychology at A level, I have found myself being able to look at the effect of the brain on our relationships and our illnesses.

It has made me appreciate how Biology and Chemistry doesn't always explain the things that we do as concisely as we're taught to believe!"

Once again give examples of how you have personally tried to achieve what you are describing.

3. **Out of the non-science subjects that you have studied, which one do you think will be useful in career in medicine and why?**

This is your opportunity to explore abstract ideas about how your favourite subjects could potentially help you to become the best doctor you could be! However, keep the weird and wonderful connections to within reason and build a solid case for the subject with 3 key points to justify why you think that subject will be useful in a medical career.

"Having studied Electronics at GSCE, I believe that it will benefit me in a future surgical career within medicine. Firstly, while learning the basic principles of building electrical circuits, the most important skill I learnt was comprehensive planning. In order to build a working circuit, all the possibilities must be thought of in advance with calculations of what capacitors; resistors and etc. are needed before a wire is laid out. This is similar to any good surgeon's routine whereby the right equipment and method must

be thought out well in advance. Secondly, in order to have a complete working circuit, vigorous testing and review of your work in progress is needed, something which every surgeon should be considering as he is carrying out any procedure. Finally, in Electronics class we were taught that although circuitry is important, presentation is equally as important in ensuring user friendliness. Similarly surgeons are always required to think about aesthetics of their finished procedure in order to satisfy patients".

4. **Out of the work experience you have done what did you enjoy the most?**

Work experience is one of the most important components of the medical student application and although it is mandatory, it should still be relatively enjoyable! Even if it was cleaning up patient faeces as a HCA, try to take any positives that you can from your work experience to be able to sell yourself, but most importantly sell the experience to the interviewers as one that has made you a better candidate to get into medical school. If you truly have had an awesome experience in your work experience, really sell it and show your enthusiasm, and as with any question, bring the example you give to life!

"My time spent working in Plaistow Hospital as a volunteer activity leader with elderly inpatients was probably the best experience from the work experience that I have done. With the activities group at the hospital, I was able to interact with such a varied and colourful group of elderly patients. This included Margaret, a former mayor of Newham who would reminisce about her time in charge while we listened to old record from the 1950s and 60s, and Rupert who was still an excellent dominos player despite being over 90 years old. It was these experiences that made me realise how important the role of the healthcare team is in ensuring that patients have a greater quality of life into their later years."

N.B. Do not use the patient's real name as this is a breech of confidentiality.

5. Tell us about your work experience?

This should be straight forward as you would have done loads and loads of different and varied work experience placements to broaden your horizons and learn a bit more about the field of medicine. Although, this would be the ideal situation; work experience in a healthcare environment has become an even more difficult goal to achieve due to the increases in health and safety regulations and increased scrutiny in healthcare environments. However, it is important that whatever work experience placement you have done, you have a clear structure for answering the question:

- Where it was: ideally in a hospital environment, although if this is not possible, just justify any location by what you gained from the experience as explained below...

- How you obtained it: Self organised placements with a good back story always show your perseverance

- What did you do: Assisting in surgery or looking after patients can look glamorous but is difficult to get to do, so working in a more administrative role may not be as fun, but can be reflected on.

- Who did you encounter? : Doctors (who can give you advice), Patients (who you enjoy spending time with and learning from) and other professionals (which helps you understand roles with the healthcare team)

- What did you learn?: This is by far the most important part of the answer, as it will show the interviewers how reflective you are as an individual and whether you have the right attitude and aptitude to be a medical student.

6. **Which of your work experience placements did you enjoy the most? What was your role there? Was it organised by your school?**

Work experience organised by yourself through determination and constant probing looks better than a scheme organised by your school every year. However, make your life easier and look out for any scheme or opportunity which is available for obtaining work experience as opportunities can be few and far between. Start looking early and if you have the opportunity to take a gap year before applying to university, don't just use it to go travelling around the world! It is an ideal chance to go to another country to do the work experience which you would never get the chance to do in this country, such as helping out in health outreach programmes.

7. What did you learn from your work experience?

Gaining some insight from your work experience is perhaps the single most important thing which interviewers are looking for in their potential medical student. They want to see that your choice in applying to do the vocation of medicine is born out of reflection and not just because "Daddy said I should be a doctor..".

Don't try to be overly dramatic i.e. "By helping the elderly, I realised I wanted to save the world from osteoporosis!". Just be realistic.

"The one thing I gained from working with the doctors at the community health centre during my time in Honduras was that medicine is about dealing with people's expectations and managing their symptoms in order for them to be able to cope with the various physical,

mental and social problems which they have. By doing this, patients are able to live happier lives and hopefully more healthy lives. My ideas about saving lives on a regular basis were somewhat crushed, however, in a way, it was saving lives, in that it was saving their quality of life eventually allowing them to live longer."

8. Have you ever raised money for charity?

Raising money for charity is a honourable thing to do, and during school there is often ample opportunity to get involved in sponsored walks, swims and rides and even book reads. Get involved! Find a charity which you identify with and help them to achieve their goals. If you have been fundraising, no matter how small an amount you were able to raise, don't be afraid to oversell your commitment to the cause. Furthermore, always try to highlight the skills gained or improved on by being involved in a fundraising activity.

"Whilst working as a volunteer at Plaistow hospital as part of the older persons activity team, I was responsible for fundraising for the activity group in order to fund the Christmas party for the inpatients. This involved coming up with ways to raise money including organising a bake sale where we sold cakes made by the volunteers to staff at the hospital, raising around £220 in total. Being responsible for the fundraising, I had to organise the volunteer

team to come up with ideas for the sale, bake the cakes and do sufficient advertising in order to attract as many staff members to the bake sale during a number of lunchtimes."

9. How do you contribute to the life of your school?

Contributing to your school life may not be easy in between studying and having a social life, however, it may not be as hard work as it sounds. Representing your school in a sport or competition, being a prefect or even mentoring younger children in your school all contribute to school life. Organising events or taking part in any clubs which happen at your school also count and despite how small it may seem, emphasise how it could have contributed to school life but also importantly what you gained from the experience apart from something to put on your CV!

"As part of my school football team, I was able to compete in the regional School's cup final at a local stadium. Being the first cup final in 7 years which any school sports team had been in, the whole of our school was invited to come down to watch after school and a couple of coaches were arranged to make this possible. It was a great day out for all involved and we eventually won 3-1. The team was honoured the next day in assembly and the atmosphere at school was fantastic for a few days. Although

we didn't change anything physical at school, we felt like we had raised the spirit of the school, with everyone from teachers to students and parents, felt a part of the victory. It was a great experience and made me realise how sport can affect lives, even at our lowly school level!"

10. How would your headmaster describe you?

You may never have personally had any dealing with your headmaster as in some schools, only the naughtiest children ever had to go to the headmaster's office, however, think about how your teachers would describe your character. Be honest and positive but also relatively professional, as more often than not your relationship with your teachers can be different to that of your friends (although this may not always be the case). Try to include examples to illustrate why they would describe you in that way based on your activities at school.

"I think that he would describe me as a pleasant, well-mannered young person who is good role model to younger students as I am currently a prefect at school. He would probably say that I'm driven, as I always like to aim for the highest marks possible, that I am athletic and a good team player as I am involved in 2 sport teams and that I am considerate as I am involved in the school's volunteering project at the local hospital."

11. You seem to have a wide variety of work experience but seem to lack work experience at a GP's practice and in hospital. Have you done anything which you have not mentioned?

This is a classic question for those who have moved heaven and earth for that work experience placement in a clinical environment and failed. Don't be disheartened! In different areas rules and regulations often make getting such placements difficult and if you are not blessed with a relative or friend who works in a clinical setting who is willing to take responsibility for you, its understandable as to why you were not able to gain a placement.

Don't be afraid to tell the interviewer how hard you have tried, and if you have got a wide range of other work experience activities they will appreciate it. The second part of this question is important however. They are looking to find out if through adversity you were able to think outside the box and gain an insight into the field of medicine by different means. This could be by going to conferences and meetings or by speaking extensively to doctors and other healthcare professionals.

"Although I haven't had the opportunity to gain work experience in a more clinical setting, I had the pleasure of being able to take part in the MedSim conference last year which was a

fantastic opportunity to gain further insight into the field of medicine. It allowed me to come to the decision that medicine is truly for me. Over the 2 day conference, I had the opportunity to take blood from a simulated arm, practise my history taking from patients as well as have a go at laparoscopic surgery. Furthermore, it was a great opportunity to meet likeminded applicants like myself but also current medical students who were able to tell me what life at medical school was really like. It was amazing and made me realise that medicine is the career path which I want to pursue."

12. You come from a college with 1500 people, do you find that daunting?

Coming from a large school or college can be difficult to make yourself standout or even feel a sense of belonging, however, it should not hold you back from anything you hope to do, and can be an advantage, helping to spur you on to be better than the rest. Being part of a big school can often mean not receiving as much help from the teacher with bigger class sizes and less special support, and so extra help can often only be available if you seek it particularly and teachers will respond if they find that their time is being appreciated.

"Being part of a large school has at times been difficult, particularly as we have quite big classes for subjects like biology and chemistry,

with sometimes 30 students usually in each class. Sometimes this can be difficult as the teachers don't get much time with us to show us some of the more difficult subjects, and when I haven't been able to understand something, I often try to go home and go over it myself. It has been a challenge, but it has meant that I have worked harder. After working through problems alone at home, I felt extremely content and was even able to help other students on the same problems which were difficult to grasp."

13. What do you currently contribute to your college?

Universities often ask this question as a way of finding out how you will contribute to their own college community if they were to give you a place. If you are currently not involved in anything which you can talk about, aim to talk about things which would look positive. Being involved with any school groups shows that you contribute to your school outside of just your education, use any experience and sell its impact regardless of how menial it may seem.

"Although I am not heavily involved in activities at my college, I do currently play football for the college representing them against other schools and colleges around the local area. It has been an invaluable experience to not only interact

with students from other institutions but also help contribute to school spirit when we are successful in our matches and able to share that success with the rest of the school population."

14. What kind of voluntary work have you done, how has it helped you?

Doing voluntary work in any sector shows that you have a caring and generous nature, as you are able to give up some of your time to help others. Volunteering can also be in your field of interest and can be something which develop your skills. This allows you to highlight the further benefit of volunteering, and talk about the things you developed as a result of your enjoyment.

"This year as part of my Duke of Edinburgh Award, I decided to volunteer as a sports assistant at a local primary school after school club. I helped teachers develop children's skills in different sports which ranged from football to cricket and basketball. Being a keen sportsman, I really enjoyed it as I got to do what I loved most, plus working with the children was so enjoyable and made the experience that much easier. Furthermore I was able to develop my teaching skills. I learnt what the best ways to show children new skills were and the teachers were really supportive and helped me develop my confidence in dealing with children in general. "

15. **You visited nursing homes for the blind, what did you do there?**

This is the kind of question that would be asked if you mentioned doing a particular activity in your personal statement. Remember that your personal statement will be the canvas by which most of your interview will be focussed on. Therefore, if you have mentioned anything in your personal statement, no matter how small a sentence, be prepared to spend some time talking about it in more detail. Just remember the general principles of talking about the experience and reflecting on what you learn and what you can take away from it.

"I did visit two different nursing homes for the blind and they were great experiences. During my time at both, I was able to spend time with both the staff and those being cared for. The staff showed me some of the challenges which they faced caring for those with disability but more importantly how they dealt with them, and it made me realise how important their jobs as carers were and how hard they work to look after those in their care. While time spent with those in the care home was enjoyable, I spent time talking and learning about living life without sight, which I found to be one of the most difficult disabilities to deal with, particularly as a vast majority of them were able to see previously. It made me realise how

important sight is and how appreciative I have to be that I am healthy. Having not had much experience with disability it was a real learning experience which I know will continue to stay with me."

16. What was the worst part of your work experience?

Depending on what you do for your work experience, it may not be as glamorous as medicine can be made to seem. Be honest with what you didn't enjoy, however, if it is something which does need to be done on a regular basis, rationalise the activity in your answer to show that you are able to reflect on the negative aspects of life.

"During my time at Plaistow hospital, I think the thing which I enjoyed the least would have to be the paperwork which I often had to help the ward clerks deal with on an everyday basis. Filing and transporting records, completing reports and entering data were all part of the job required of me during the placement which sometimes made my time there long and tedious, with not as much medical experience gained as I would have liked. Despite this, the work I was doing was clearly invaluable to the work done by the doctors and nurses, as effective record-keeping is an essential part of providing good patient care and I often saw how much paperwork some of the junior

doctors had to do as part of their everyday work, such as discharge summaries, which must have been just as tedious but even more important."

17. Do you remember any particular patient that did not have a good outcome?

This could be a talking point for further questions particularly if they were suffering from a treatable medical condition, such as what the condition was and what other options might have been available. While on work experience, take interest in the patients, and if you don't know about any conditions, don't be afraid to ask, and find out about what the medical team can do to help them. This shows your inquisitive nature, but more importantly as a doctor, your patients are your job and are your responsibility so you must be able to take a keen interest in them.

"One patient I particularly remember was Margaret, a former mayor of Plaistow who was a very pleasant lady. Unfortunately, while in hospital she had a bad pneumonia which left her very weak. It was not responding to antibiotics and after her sputum was cultured, the doctors discovered that it was an MRSA-pneumonia. Despite changing her antibiotics and the best efforts of the medical team, she wasn't able to pull through and she passed away. It was quite sad, as she was loved on the

ward. It showed how susceptible patients are while in hospital to even the rarer complications of being in hospital."

N.B. Do not use the patient's real name as this is a breech of confidentiality.

18. **Did you see any patients that had a good outcome?**

Seeing a patient get through a difficult illness is something which every doctor takes heart from. When describing the scenario, don't be afraid of highlighting exactly what you think contributed to the good outcome, whether it was medical intervention, care from the nurses, love from the patient's family or the patient's own will and inner strength.

"One patient I saw at the hospital who made a great recovery was a man called Albert. He had a stroke and had been in hospital for some months being unable to talk or walk. He then suffered from pneumonia and the doctors didn't think that he would be able to survive another 2 weeks. Even his daughter was warned of the implications. However, he had 3 grandchildren who came to visit on a regular basis and he recovered from the pneumonia, and soon started to work on his rehabilitation. He was able to start make sounds and talking within a month with help of a speech therapist and the physiotherapists who worked hard to get him using a Zimmer frame. It was great to see and it

showed the hard work done by other healthcare professionals apart from doctors."

19. **What steps have you taken to learn more about medicine?**

There are many resources and methods of finding out more about medicine which you can discuss in a question such as this. To start with, your work experience is the first and most valuable resource. If taken in an environment involving the care of doctors, you can gain as much from just being there and observing how they work as well as asking them personally about the job that they do. Reading journals, articles and websites can also be good to gain an insight into the knowledge base of medicine, learning more about what advances have been made in the field and what is within the scope of the medical field. Going to conferences and meetings, can allow you to network with a group of medical professionals and like-minded individuals in a certain field. Remember that the more you do, the more you can talk about.

When talking about your experiences, give specifics about where and when you did them and signpost what you have learned from your experience so that the interviewer knows that it wasn't a wasted opportunity. Also feel free to reflect on the experience, maybe how it could have been improved. However be careful not to criticise!

" One of the steps I took to learn more about medicine this year was to attend the Medisix conference in Nottingham. The conference had a range of lectures focussed on the medical profession, with prominent speakers talking about their fields."

20. **What is your greatest achievement you have attained thus far in your education?**

Being the high flyer which you obviously are since you are reading this, it shouldn't be too hard talking about your greatest academic achievement. When outlining any achievement, think STAR: Situation, task, achievement and reflection. Start by putting your achievement into context by giving a background of the circumstances surrounding it, perhaps a difficult time in your life, or it was previously your weakest subject or area. Follow by explaining the tasks which you undertook to achieve, such as the extra work you did. Then talk about what you achieved and summarise by reflecting on what you learn throughout the process of getting there.

"I think my greatest achievement in my education so far was getting the highest mark in my class for my C1 and C2 papers in AS Maths. After getting a B in GCSE Maths, a subject which I really enjoyed, I was determined to improve my performance for my A-levels. As

soon as we received our textbooks for C1 and C2

I systematically went through at least 1 chapter

a week regardless of the work we were doing in

class which included doing extra questions from

a maths question book donated by a family

friend. I set aside 3 hours just for extra Maths

work a week apart from my homework. We

took C1 in January and C2 in June and I got the

highest marks in the class for both. It showed

that if I put in the hours and the work in

anything, I can improve and be the best I can

be. I was quite proud of myself and have used it

as inspiration to try to improve my chemistry A-

levels grades in A2."

21. **What in the history of medicine has really interested you?**

If a particular discovery or aspect of medical history has captured your imagination, make sure you know the facts before you start talking about it, as it is most likely that the interviewers will be medical professionals, and they may have knowledge of the advancement you are talking about. Ideally your interest in a particular historical event would be because of a possible interest in the medical speciality where it happened.

OR If you want to try and suck up to your potential medical school, talk about the medical advancements which they have been involved with in the past, such as the discovery of DNA for King's or the formation of Gray's anatomy textbook at St Georges!

Remember to comment on why it has sparked your interest and the lessons that can be learned from the event.

"I think what interested me the most in the history of medicine, has to be the discovery of anaesthesia in the 1800s which allowed the field of surgery to progress into what is today, while being an example of the sacrifices made by doctors to further the field of medicine. Starting with Humphrey Davy trying nitrous oxide and nicknaming it laughing gas because of its effect, to the first public demonstration of an anaesthetic agent by William Morton, it

changed the face of surgery. It allowed surgeons to develop newer more explorative procedures now that pain was eliminated. Often the early discoverers of anaesthetics had to try these agents on themselves or close friends in order to make the discoveries which is shows the sacrifice they were willing to make. For me as someone who would love to be a surgeon, their sacrifices have allowed surgery to continue to breakdown boundaries in saving lives."

22. What impressed you most about the doctors in your work experience?

During your work experience, you would have hopefully seen doctors in action in their everyday jobs. It is not always as glamorous as TV would make it seem, however, there is a hope that during your time in work experience you will observe common traits and themes in what being a doctor is all about and what the job entails. When answering this question, think about the a character trait or job which you saw most commonly and then describe and reflect on it.

"Whilst working with some of the doctors at Plaistow Hospital, one of the things which impressed me the most was the ability for the doctors to remain calm in a variety of situations. Whether it was dealing with a cardiac arrest, trying to get an agitated inpatient back into bed, or talking to frustrated relatives, everyday tested the patience of the doctors who worked in the hospital in different *ways. It is something which I truly admired and hope that if I get the opportunity to study medicine, I will be able to exhibit my patience in the same manner."*

23. **Describe a difficult situation you have dealt with in your work experience and what did you learn from it?**

During your work experience you are unlikely to handle patients yourself or deal with difficult clinical decisions. You are more likely to be faced with emotional dilemmas which you may not have faced before. These present a great opportunity to display your morality and discuss any growth in your character.

"During my work experience at Plaistow Hospital,

I was fortunate to be allowed to spend time on the wards, helping the ward clerks and doctors in minor tasks. I didn't face many demanding situations, however, the most difficult situation was witnessing a ward doctor breaking bad news to the family of one of the inpatient's who had just passed away. Having spent quite a lot of time with the patient I was invited to support the doctor in delivering the news. I found it difficult mainly because it was so disappointing and uncomfortable to deliver such bad news to the family and see their reaction. It made me realise firstly that death is inevitably a part of life, but more importantly, that because of that fact, it is part of a doctor's job to support the patient and their family in death. Being sensitive to the *family's mood and being empathetic are a key*

part to breaking bad news, attributes which I

believe I have, but I think death is something

which I shall have get used to."

24. Have you ever been in a position of responsibility and something went wrong?

This is similar to the question on responsibility, however, for this question focus on how you dealt with failure and used initiative to fix the problem. Choose a simple example, explain what your responsibility was, what went wrong and why, any attempts to fix the mistake, what you learnt, what you could improve on next time, and most importantly how you can apply this lesson to medical practice.

Industry based Questions

1. Do you think pharmacists are sometimes tempted to advise a customer to buy an expensive product even if there is a cheaper one available?

This is a circumstantial question so you have to weigh up both arguments for and against even if you believe, and perhaps know what the answer is, you cannot afford to generalise. Be honest with yourself and the interviewer if you lack a perspective, as this shows your honesty and if possible, offer to try and improve yourself by wanting to find out. Also, feel free to provide your own personal commentary as long as you distinguish it as your own opinion.

"I think that there may be some pharmacists, who are tempted to sell more expensive products, particularly if they stand to make a profit directly from its sale, but hopefully, those products may also be of better or more proven quality and so the sale of it is still justified. I think that a problem with commercialising healthcare will always cause dilemmas such as this, as when should the healthcare provider stop being a seller and vice versa. I don't know if pharmacists have the same duty to their

patients as doctors do, however, it would be

nice to know that pharmacists care about the

wellbeing of their customers and would not just

sell products to make money, but also ensure

that they are doing the best for their health."

THE HUMAN GENOME PROJECT

2. How will the Human Genome project help treat patients in the future?

The Human Genome project is a international scientific research project with the primary goal of determining the sequence of the DNA in order to identify and map the 25,000 genes which make up the human genome. By doing so, it will be possible to find genes that cause disease and possibly use the information to develop more specific treatments. This allows us to open up the field of genetic medicine, and in the near future be able to modify genes in order to prevent diseases from occurring in humans. Pre-implantation genetic diagnosis is used to prevent children with life-affecting illnesses from being born, while genetic tests for conditions such as breast cancer can help to manage patients early on and prevent disease. Furthermore, all the information and research found by the HGP is freely available allowing the scientific community to continue their research into genes that causes disease.

"I think that the HGP is important for furthering research into the diagnosis, treatment and

prevention of diseases in patients both today and in the future. The ability to screen patients for genes that make them susceptible to disease such as the BRCA1 gene for breast cancer has saved thousands of lives. Surely there must be many more conditions which genetic testing can continue to help influence and save lives. The fact that it has remained a free to use resource means that scientists can continue to use the information to progress their research and this will hopefully help build more specific genetic treatments to accompany the advances in diagnoses that have been made!"

3. **What are the advantages and disadvantages to 'The Human Genome Project'?**

There are many advantages to the Human Genome Project which has allowed it to become one of the most important scientific discoveries of recent times. Firstly, it has allowed us to revolutionise the way that we diagnose, treat and even prevent many conditions which affect human beings. People can be offered genetic testing for a number of illnesses which can show predisposition in the genome such as breast cancer, clotting disorders and liver disease, while at the same time genetic testing can be used to screen embryos for more life-affecting conditions such as Huntington's disease or cystic fibrosis. Secondly, the HGP has allowed us to further understand human biology and its relation to the other organisms in the world. Through the project it was seen that only 7% of our genes differentiate us from other vertebrate animals. It has allowed the scientific community to better understand the evolution process as well as understanding key cellular processes which occur in our bodies every second. Despite this, here are some disadvantages to having access to such information, and it mainly revolves around the ethical dilemmas that the HGP poses. The prospect of "designer babies" continues to loom, as the ability to carry out pre-implantation genetic diagnosis allows parents to screen out diseases, but could in the future be used to target certain genes for the better, such as intelligence, strength and body type. Furthermore, the use of the HGP to study populations has been criticised as the study of an ethnic group's genome which is carried out without their consent and therefore, it is thought to be unethical.

In your answer, knowledge of the key advantages and disadvantages would be sufficient. The most important point about your answer to the question is making sure it is succinct. Give the main points, with a short example for each, and tie it together with your own summary.

"I believe that the HGP is a key asset in the development of new diagnostic tools, innovative

treatments and preventative methods for many of the illnesses which affect human beings. For example, genetic tests can be offered to people with susceptibility to breast cancer, looking for the BRCA 1 gene allows doctors to remove a woman's breast as a preventative measure to avoid an early death from the disease. Furthermore, it has helped us to understand human biology, with the HGP giving us new information on the central role played by DNA in the determining cellular processes.

The greater knowledge is invaluable but it also means that it can be abused, and I know that "designer babies" are one way by which knowledge of the human genome can be *dangerous if not adequately controlled. Despite this, I believe the opportunities created by the HGP has changed medicine for the better and hope we can continue to use it for the benefit of curing and preventing disease. "*

4. **What sort of laws should be passed on to prevent people taking advantages over The Human Genome Project?**

This is a difficult question as there are a whole host of answers which you can give! Feel free to offer your opinion (not too strongly), focus in on a specific aspect of the HGP which could be an issue. The biggest concern for the HGP is what the information is going to be used for, and how it could be used. "Designer babies" in which parents could chose certain genetic traits using IVF pre-implantation techniques are probably the most ethically and morally controversial area which comes out of the HGP. Laws which limit its use in creating new human beings could be used to prevent such action.

"Although I know very little about law and what laws could be passed, I believe that any law which prevented people from creating new human beings by tampering with their DNA would be the most important one to stop people taking advantage of the information provided by the HGP. I think that the ability to create human life by selecting favourable genes is ethically wrong and should not be allowed as it

exploits the breakthrough of pre-implantation genetic diagnosis."

NHS PROBLEMS

5. Have there been any dramatic changes to the NHS since it was founded?

The NHS has not changed in its principles since it was founded in 1948. Care is still free at point of use, except for prescriptions and dental charges, everyone is eligible for care (even visitors to the UK), and it is funded by government collected taxes. It is still based on the system of the GP being the "gatekeeper" to hospital services, and hospitals being run by regional organisations.

What has changed is the way in which the system is run. Originally run as a giant organisation, a culture of an internal market was formed in the 1990 NHS and Community Care Act. This meant that local authorities and some GPs would be able to act as buyers of services from hospitals and other organisations, in the hope that this would increase competition and raise standards. The new Health and Social Care bill passed in 2012 is the greatest threat to the fundamental structure of the NHS. By abolishing the regional organisations that run hospitals, and giving more power to GPs to buy services from hospitals. This makes hospitals more vulnerable to competition and could lead the way for a more privatised healthcare system. Read more about the short history of the NHS at www.nhshistory.net

"I think that the values of the NHS remain the same since it was founded in 1x948, which is to provide free tax-paid healthcare to all. In recent times, the emphasis on patient satisfaction has been pushed to the forefront, which I believe is important, however, the new healthcare improvements put in place are the most dramatic changes to the NHS. It abolishes the regional healthcare authorities responsible for

the hospitals and replaces them with GP run organisations. This move presents the greatest change in NHS culture as local health authorities were established with the founding of the NHS, but it also makes GPs more responsible for the financial burden of healthcare, which poses its own ethical dilemmas."

6. **Did you know your local health authority has the largest number of bed blockers? How should the NHS go about removing bed blockers?**

Bed blocking is when elderly patients cannot be discharged due a lack of care homes places or home help adaptations. This is a major problem in the UK with serious cuts in social care which means that many older people are not receiving the support they require to stay healthy and out of hospitals, leading to a rise in the number of readmissions and A&E visits from elderly people. With the country and more importantly the NHS in a time of cutbacks, it is vital that bed-blocking is dealt with, in order to save both money and resources.

So how should it be dealt with? One recent report from the London School of Economics found £625 million of taxpayers' money could be saved if more stair lifts and handrails were installed in people's homes allowing them to stay independent for longer. However, should the NHS be responsible for ensuring elderly people are kitted out in their homes?

Feel free to express possible ideas to these sorts of questions, as long as they are relatively reasonable i.e. not "kick 'em out of their beds!".

"I didn't know that my local health authority had the largest number of bed blockers, but I do recognise that bed blocking is a national problem. This means that many NHS hospitals are losing money due to it, particularly in a time where cuts have to be made. I think one of the main problems is the lack of social care provision and possibly inadequate communication between NHS hospitals and

their local social care organisation. I think what the NHS itself could do is help its healthcare professionals improve the discharge and follow up planning to prevent re-admission into hospital."

7. What is wrong with the NHS?

One could spend an entire day answering this question. However, what is currently wrong with the NHS is that there is not enough money in the system. What is the reason? As most clinicians will tell you, it is because it is almost impossible to count the cost of illness. One patient's pneumonia could take 3 weeks to clear, while another, just one week. This results in an extra 2 weeks which cannot be price-coded in the same way. Similarly another person's appendectomy could take an hour long than the next, resulting in having to pay staff one more hour of wage in order to complete the operation. Across the NHS, inability to account for the unexpected nature of illness means that attempts to treat all patients equally and fairly undermines the values of running a cost effective service. However despite this, there are ways to save money while making services efficient enough to deal with patients, and this is what the NHS needs to focus on. The NHS needs to cut unnecessary management costs in order to re-organise and re-shape its services to where they are needed the most.

If you choose to focus on a particular area of the NHS, ensure you know a bit about the problem so that you can be prepared if asked to discuss it in more detail.

"The NHS has many problems, and as an outsider, I couldn't really make a judgement on what is wrong with the NHS itself. However, I do believe that the nature of the business in dealing with unexpected illness makes it vulnerable to the costing of that illness. There is no way to be able to budget for procedures and treatments for different patients, as there could be a large difference in cost for the same illness. Its not the same as a consumer based system,

where the customer asks for what they want and when they get it, they are happy. The NHS deals in making people well, and as long as the treatment is covered by NHS guidelines, it means that for as long as it takes, treatment will be given until deemed not in the patient's best interest, and this could cost much more than expected. I think this is one of the reasons that the NHS have a big financial problem."

8. What does the World Health Organisation do?

The World Health Organisation (WHO) is a specialist department of the United Nations (UN) which deals with international public health. Founded in 1948, it was charged with improving public health across the globe to allow people to attain the highest possible level of health, particularly in the fields of communicable and sexually transmitted diseases as well to improve maternal and child health. Its major triumph as a organisation has been its leading role in the eradication of small pox, while currently it leads the way in fighting HIV/AIDS around the world as part of the UNAIDS network. The two other major communicable diseases which it aims to combat is malaria and tuberculosis.

Learn more about the WHO and some of its success stories from the WHO website. www.who.int

"I know that the World Health Organisation is an UN organisation responsible for international public health. It produces the World Health Report which is a leading publication on health and also organises the World Health Day. I know that it produces many reports on the health status of various diseases as well as working to reduce the effect of communicable diseases on populations around the world. Recently, work on reducing congenital rubella syndrome in children by introducing measles and rubella vaccines in initiatives around the developing world has been extremely successful, with WHO plans to eliminate measles and rubella in more than 80% of the world by 2020."

9. **If you were the head of a group of doctors and a colleague was not doing the job well, what would you do?**

    Think about how you would respond to a team member that was not pulling their weight. Although there is technically no right answer, the interviewer wants to know that you will be able to deal with people in a team environment in an appropriate manner.

    Remember that giving a team member the opportunity to improve by first offering feedback is often the first line of helping to improve performance within a team.

"As the head of the group, I would look to understand why my colleague was not doing their job appropriately. This would involve a personal consultation with the team member finding out if they had any particular problems and offer support if they did. I would also highlight any deficiencies which I would suggest they could improve on. We could then review things after a time period in order to monitor how things were progressing. If there were no improvements, this would result in thinking about more serious implications for the involved parties if needed."

10. **If you were asked to design four stamps to mark the 50th anniversary of the NHS, what would you put on the stamps and why?**

"The stamp designs which I would choose would be:

- *The iconic blue and white NHS logo – this is because it is an instantly recognisable logo associated with all things associated with healthcare in this country. Every building, vehicle, and paraphernalia linked to the NHS is branded with the logo, and could work well if presented in a different colour to the regular blue and white.*

- *A picture of doctors and nurses at work – as these professions are the backbone of the NHS it would make sense to show them at work in a hospital environment.*

- *A portrait picture of Aneurin Bevan – He was the health minister in 1948 who unveiled the dream of bringing good healthcare to all financed by central taxation. As the "founding father" of the NHS it would be appropriate to honour him though a postage stamp.*

- *A picture of some backroom staff such as porters, cleaners and administrators – to highlight that the NHS needs all these people in order for it to run as effective as it does. "*

11. **If you where the prime minister what three government policies would you set to achieve?**

Think of sensible achievable policies which are currently being employed and think of ways in which you could improve them. This can be a detailed answer if need be, however, think of trying to summarise the key points of the policies which you would focus on.

"As prime minister I would focus on government policies which would improve healthcare but through less direct means.

- *I focus on healthcare organisation and efficient running of NHS hospitals in order to reduce deficits*

- *I would improve provision for social care in order to ensure there were enough resources to look after the elderly, particularly those who are more vulnerable. This would reduce bed-blocking.*

- *Finally, I would invest in public health initiatives such as increasing exercise and eating more healthily to continue to improve the general health of the nation. Problems such as obesity, diabetes and hypertension are preventable and is key to reducing the cost of treatments."*

12. Give me three extended roles of nurses in the modern healthcare system?

In the modern healthcare system, the role of the nurse has been extended for a number of reasons. Demand on the remit of the doctor means that more responsibility shared with other healthcare professionals means more efficient use of time, while more educated and engaged nurses allows for better care for the patients.

Nurse practitioners are nurses with an increased role within the healthcare team:

- They are able to diagnose, treat and evaluate patients with acute and chronic illness and disease such as asthma or diabetes

- They can prescribe drugs

- Order and perform diagnostic tests

- Obtain medical histories and carry out medical examinations

Being able to spend time with nurse practitioner during your work experience would be an invaluable time spent as they can carry out many tasks which doctors do on a regular basis.

"I know that nurses in the modern healthcare system can now become nurse practitioners who have more responsibility and knowledge which allows them to deal with patients often without help from a doctor. They are often specialised in a particular field such as asthma. I know that they are able to take medical histories and examinations in order to help diagnose, prescribe treatments and manage patients and their conditions. I think this is invaluable to the NHS as it allows doctors to focus on other things, such as managing more difficult patients, and means that nurses can contribute more to the healthcare environment".

13. How do you think the health system should be funded? Give me your opinion.

As this questions asks for your opinion, you are entitled to say whatever you feel as long as you can justify why you have said it. There is on right or wrong answer as explained previously. However, have a good structure to your answer as always, think about what the problem currently is, what you are suggesting, why you are suggesting it and how it could be achieved.

"I believe that the funding of the health system is currently inadequate and taken advantage of by individuals as they feel that it is their right to expect treatment regardless of cost, despite their contribution to tax-paying. Although it is a good principle, I think the NHS should be semi-privatised, so that each person is given a certain budget and if their treatments exceed this, they will have to pay the remainder. This would reduce the amount of people who abuse the health service with minor ailments, but also means that care would be improved as more money would be available for improving the semi-privatised services."

14. European Working Directive - what do you know about them?

The European Working Time Directive is a law passed by the European Union which must be followed by its member states, of which the

United Kingdom is one. It entitles each worker to have:

- a minimum of 20 days of leave in a full time job
- a daily rest of 11 hours in a 24 hour period
- no more than 48 hours working in a 7 day period

This has had huge implications on the shift patterns of doctors as it means that on-call shifts have effectively been shortened to no longer than 12 hours. However, in the UK it is possible to opt out of the 48 hour week rule and work longer hours. Some may see it as a step forward in protecting patients from tired, over-worked doctors, but many clinicians have felt that it often means that junior doctors lack the experience of being in hospital which helps them become better doctors.

"I know that the European Working Time Directive is a EU law which has changed the working patterns of doctors, particularly junior doctors in the UK, restricting them to 48 hour weeks and no longer than 12 hour days. Although this makes for less tired and stressed doctors, it also has any implication on staffing and the level of exposure for junior doctors as they are in hospital much less than before."

15. What do you believe should be the uniform for doctors in these modern times?

Hospital trusts vary across the UK in what constitutes the appropriate dress code. While some favour smart clothing, others believe in wearing surgical scrubs or specialised uniforms. White coats were a big no-no a few years ago, however, white tunics have now been adopted by trusts such as Guys and St Thomas'.

What is most important however, is that whatever uniform a doctor wears, it does not impede on their ability to carry out their role, both physically but also perceptually, and that it is suitably able to reduce the risk of infection control.

"I believe that any uniform that is firstly, suitably adapted to prevent the spread of infection, such as short sleeves and a clean clear colour, and secondly, is appropriate for the hospital environment, both for the doctor and for patients, is acceptable. I think that scrubs are a good choice, and they make the HCP stand out from visitors and could be colour coded or named to even identify different healthcare professionals."

16. Is the Hippocratic Oath still relevant today?

The Hippocratic Oath was thought to be written by Hippocrates who was considered the father of western medicine. It outlines some of the duties of a doctor to his patients and serves as a moral code for doctors to follow. The BMA made a Revised Hippocratic Oath which outlines a more up to date version, something which can also be found at the front of the Oxford Clinical Handbook of Medicine. Make sure you read the full Oath if you get the chance to and apply it to any ethical dilemmas asked to discuss in your interview. Whether it is still relevant today is a matter for discussion. One of the statements within the oath includes: "I will not put profit or my own career above my duty to my patient", which in a healthcare system outside the NHS is something which can be difficult to keep to. However, in the free to access healthcare such as the NHS, doctors are can freely look after their patients without thinking about profit.

"I believe that the Hippocratic Oath is still relevant today. I think that doctors do abide by the principles outlined in the oath, such as using your knowledge for good, and each patient's health is the doctor's primary concern. One of the more controversial aspects of the Oath which conflicts with some of the paid healthcare systems is that "I will not put profit ... above my duty to my patient". Outside the NHS, in healthcare systems where money plays a big part of the treatment plan, it can be difficult to uphold the Oath when it affects the amount of money you will earn as a doctor. However, I still have faith in the medical profession and believe thousands of doctors around the world are doing the best for their patients."

17. Who are the General Medical Council?

The General Medical Council is an organisation which is responsible for keeping a register of the medical practitioners licensed within the public sector in Britain. It also regulates medical schools in the UK and sets the standards of professional and ethical practice.

It is important to have a regulatory body free from governmental control and it is vital to making sure that doctors are operating within adequate boundaries.

"The General Medical Council are the main regulatory body for doctors, and are responsible for keeping a list of doctors licensed to practice medicine in the UK as well as setting the professional standards for doctors. I know that they are also responsible for overseeing medical education and regulating UK medical schools. I think that this is vital to ensure that doctors uphold certain standards and that the public are protected."

18. Who are the Medicines and Healthcare products Regulatory Agency (MHRA)?

The Medicines and Healthcare Products Regulatory Agency (MHRA) is a government organisation responsible for ensuring that medicines and medical devices work and are acceptably safe. It is responsible for monitoring adverse drug reactions to medicines and incidents with medical devices as well as making sure that drugs and devices comply with regulation.

"The MHRA are a government agency responsible for ensuring medicines and medical devices work and are safe. Their main responsibility is reporting, investigating and monitoring of adverse drug reactions to medicines and incidents with medical devices. As well as this, they ensure both drugs and devices comply to regulation and regulate clinical trials of both. This is a vital function in healthcare as drugs and devices are by far the most common methods of treating and managing patients."

19. What is holistic medicine?

Holistic medicine is a method of looking at medicine which upholds all the aspects of people's needs, including the psychological, physical and social aspects. This is thought to be a widely held view in treating patients in modern medicine. Practices undertaken in holistic medicine include natural diets and herbal remedies, nutritional supplements, psycho-spiritual counselling, acupuncture and homeopathy. Although this method often seems to please many patients as the treatments are more personalised; there is no published scientific studies which prove the efficacy of holistic medicine past the placebo effect on any known disease.

"Holistic medicine is a concept in medicine which looks at the psychological, physical and social aspect of the patient and taking them all into account. Some of the practices included in holistic medicine include homeopathy, acupuncture and natural herbal remedies, which can often be personalised to the patient. This is therefore thought to cause a placebo effect in terms of treating disease, as there is no

published scientific data on the efficacy of holistic medicine practices."

20. In your opinion, where do you see the health service going?

With the new NHS healthcare bill being approved, the NHS could go in a number of directions. One which has particularly concerned many observers is the fact that more power is going to GP consortia and increasing internal competition. This will cause a shift towards patients having to pay for certain services which could eventually lead to a fully privatised healthcare service. Feel fee to express your opinion if they ask, as long as it's reasonable.

"I think that with the introduction of the new Healthcare Bill which sees greater power going to GPs in the form of consortia and a greater emphasis on internal competition, this leaves the NHS open to new challenges. The main one would be preventing new private competitors from taking patients away from NHS hospitals thus weakening the health system, and eventually leading to the rise of private hospitals. This could lead to a semi-privatised system, whereby patients would have to pay for certain services, and in the long term, to a fully privatised insurance based health system similar to the US."

21. Do you read newspapers? Name an interesting medical related story.

Reading daily or weekly newspapers is important to your own personal development in making sure that you are up-to-date with current issues as well as taking in well written opinions about what is going on in the world. Any publications are good enough, and with the emergence of tablet PCs, often publications are available electronically. Make sure you have read though a number of current magazines or newspapers which you can talk about at your interview. Always try to reflect on the piece that you have read, in order to show that you have insight into a particular topic.

"I usually like to read the Daily Telegraph as well as The Times as my regular newspapers. One article in the Telegraph which caught my eye was the recent discovery that giving immunoglobulins in the early part of Alzheimer's disease could potentially prevent the mental decline in patients by up to 3 years. With our ever aging population with more and more people living longer, Alzheimer's disease will become a huge burden on people and the economy. It is good that there is plenty of research being done in this field to prevent Alzheimer's becoming a major issue in the world. "

22. How do you go about keeping up-to-date with current medical issues?

This question is asking how you show your interest in the field of medicine through reading, and it is important to show that you do so via a variety of reliable methods. Always be prepared to talk about a current article you may have seen from the sources you mentioned.

- Newspapers, although good for reading, lack concrete scientific grounding, often paraphrasing from real science to fit their purpose.

- Magazines such as the New Scientist are well rounded scientific publications which help broaden your knowledge of science around the world.

- The internet is the main source of information in the world today, many websites have health sections such as the BBC, while you can search for numerous scientific journals and abstracts in the fields which you are interested in.

"I usually keep up to date with current medical issues via a number of different ways. I try to keep up daily by visiting a website called medicalnewstoday.com which collates sources from a variety of journals such as the BMJ and JAMA as well as other news sources to deliver medical news. It is usually the first place I look for and read about developments in medicine, while I also use the BBC Health website to look

at more British focused news articles. Furthermore, I subscribe to the New Scientist magazine, which I find to be a really good read, updating me on current medical and scientific news while having a range of interesting articles."

23. What do you read of a medical nature?

Reading more specific journals and medical magazines highlights a more direct interest in the field of medicine. The student British Medical Journal for example, are great entry level journals for students to read.

"I like to read the student British Medical Journal which has a range of interesting articles, including tips for in medical school and ways to improve studying and learning. In addition to this, it keeps me up to date with developments in the medical world both in the UK and abroad. I thoroughly enjoy the way that it is written and hope to continue to subscribe to it if I get into medical school."

24. Tell us about any medical articles you have seen in the media recently?

Like mentioned before, always be prepared to talk about a few medical articles which have recently been in the news, as they will be expecting you to know about the biggest stories. Reflect on the news article and put it into context.

"One interesting article, I read on the BBC News health website recently discussed the risks of moderate drinking on the risk of dementia. A longitudinal study in the US showed that women in their 60s who drank a moderate amount of alcohol, around 7-14 units of alcohol a week, increased their risk of developing problems with memory and brain functioning. They also found that fortnightly binges also increase the risk of dementia like symptoms in both men and women. I believe that if the research has some truth, this could have huge implications on future generations of Britons

given our "binge drinking" culture and a substantial rise in women drinking much higher quantities of alcohol."

25. What do you believe has been the biggest recent breakthrough in medicine recently?

There are hundreds of new advances in medicine happening each year, by keeping well-informed of the latest medical news, you will be able to talk about one which has interested you enough to believe that it has been the biggest. This is another opinion question and so as long as you can justify why you think it is the biggest breakthrough then your answer will receive an A*.

"I believe one of the biggest breakthroughs in medicine has to be the new totally artificial heart which is now being fitted in patients around the world. These hearts can replace both ventricles of a patient's failing heart and allow them to be able to lead a better quality of life whilst waiting for a donor heart. I believe that this is revolutionary as it allows many patients to have a new lease of life during their wait for a donor heart, which can often be a long process. With 1000 artificial hearts already fitted, perhaps in the near future it may be secure and safe enough to be able to use on a more long term basis and perhaps reduce the need for heart transplants."

26. What was the last book/article I read about medicine?

Reading medicine related books, may be slightly premature as you may not have a place in medical school, but be positive and don't be afraid to see what doctors are reading in order to align your mind frame early. Reading books which may give you an insight into the medical career are definitely more useful at this stage of your education to help you make a more informed decision about medicine.

"The last medical related book I read was a book by Dr Riaz Agha called "Making Sense of Your Medical Career". It was a book which I

found at a family friend's house which I thought may be an interesting read in allowing me to understand more about the medical career path. It was quite simple and easy to read and talked about some of the key things which you should be doing while at medical school and early in your career, to ensure that you are on track in making it to the top. I would recommend it to all young medical professionals and students. "

27. **What major issue are currently affecting the NHS?**

The NHS are affected by a number of issues, and the news agencies in the UK do not fail to highlight them, with almost a news article a day commenting on the NHS. Keep up-to-date with any current scandals or long running problems by reading more topical news articles and websites such as the BBC Health website.

"I know that the major issue facing the NHS currently is its financial management, particularly in this time of austerity. In the news, there has been recent articles relating to the massive debts faced by the South London Healthcare Trust which puts 5 major South London hospitals in danger of closing some departments or even whole sites. It is due to be put into administration which is a worrying prospect as there must be hundreds to thousands of people who rely on those

hospitals, and if any were to close, it would

have a significant impact on the entire region."

28. How do you think doctors are viewed in the current media?

Negative high profile stories about doctors are always going to be around as the media always focus on the negatives and less on the positives particularly in professions or fields where they feel people are highly paid compared to the general population. Use this question to demonstrate your knowledge of recent medical stories which involve doctors; this will impress your interviewer(s).

"I think that the current media viewpoint of

doctors is not currently positive, especially as they often like to focus on the stories of individual doctors who may not be doing good things. I read a recent Telegraph article on the internet about a consultant who in the recent doctor's strike, cancelled his NHS clinic due to strike action, but was not too far away doing paid work at a private hospital. Stories like that affect public confidence in doctors, and with high profile stories such as Harold Shipman and Andrew Wakefield, it seems that the media will take any opportunity to bring down the medical profession. Despite this, I think the one medium which is very sympathetic to doctors is television, with programmes like 24hours in A&E and Junior Doctors."

29. What do you consider to be important advances in medicine over the last 50 years?

"I believe that one of the most important advances in medicine over the last 50 years has to be the completion of the Human Genome Project which has opened a new chapter in the treatment of genetic diseases. It has also helped the treatment of conditions such as diabetes and hypertension which have certain predisposing genes that can now be identified and studied in more closely. It has revolutionised the way that we diagnose, treat and manage patients with genetically linked diseases as well allowed the medical world to create simple and effective screening tools to

prevent certain diseases manifesting. I think that superior knowledge of our genome is vital in the development of better treatments and understanding of diseases where little is known; this will continue to help the field of medicine grow."

30. How do you think the rise in technology has influenced and will continue to influence the practice of medicine?

Technological advances go hand in hand with medical advances and are needed in order for doctors to be able to test the boundaries of medicine in a safe and secure manner. Technology allows information to be processed quicker than we as humans can manage, as well as being the backbone for newer more efficient imaging techniques, diagnostic tools and reporting of results. The switch from paper to electronic records is also vital in making sure patient care can be monitored more closely and information shared amongst healthcare teams is much quicker. Give some examples of the technological success stories which are driving medicine.

"I think that the rise in technology is the most important factor in influencing how medicine is now practised in the developed world. The advancement of computers means that better imaging techniques such as MRI and CT can be used. There are always new programs being *developed for these. It also allows more and more information to be processed electronically, such as patient records, results and managing patient treatment plans. Even in surgery, robots allow surgeons to be more precise in their operations, reducing human unsteadiness and error. The internet also allows the instant transfer of information both for learning and treating patients; this means that doctors around the world are more informed about medicine in general. I believe that this will continue to drive the medical field in the future and that nearly all of the medicine which doctors practice will require some sort of technology."*

31. What social factors can affect people seeking medical help?

"Due to beliefs about the meaning of poor health in some cultures, e.g. a punishment from God, they are less willing to ask for help and pride may also play a role. In the elderly, the lack of a support system whilst living alone may prevent them from asking for help with anyone to prompt them. Some may not be able to afford prescriptions and transport to the G.P. or hospital whilst others may be not be able to take time off work and visit the G.P. during their working day."

32. What is the role of the minister of health?

This question will get you points if you know the precise answer:

"The health minister is also known as the secretary of state for health. It is his role to promote public health, and make decisions regarding healthcare budget distribution."

Your view on becoming a doctor based questions

1. **What is your impression of the job of a doctor?**

"A doctors role is multi-faceted. Doctors are healers, communicators, counselors, educators, facilitators and leaders. Each part is almost as important as the other in saving and preserving life, which is the overall goal of doctors. Being able to carry out a life saving procedure is just as important as educating a patient on their

care, as well as being supportive to their needs or even leading an efficient healthcare team to look after the patient. In your answer, remember that being a doctor is more than just saving people from life threatening illness, it is also about managing their expectations, both physically and mentally, in order to bring about better health."

2. Do you think doctors just work from 9am-5pm?

If you thought doctors worked just 9-5, you would be highly misinformed. It was only until recently, junior doctors would work long on-call shifts, often being in hospital for around 48 hours at a time to cover ward shifts and then have less than a day off before being back at work. Even GPs were expected to be on call 24hrs, 7 days a week, as part of their service to their patients. Although the European Working Time Directive has changed all of this, many junior doctors still have to work past their registered hours in order to make sure patients are cared for adequately. On call shifts are still compulsory although now usually around 12 hours long.

"I don't think the job of a doctor is as straightforward as 9-5, especially as people can get sick at any time and therefore it is probably one of the more unpredictable jobs, in terms of when you are needed. It wouldn't make sense

for doctors to stop working after 5pm as it would mean so many people would suffer as a result of no cover, particularly specialists for the night time hours which can be the busiest times for presenting to hospital. Furthermore, in order to be able to deal with situations and emergencies which can arise with patients being treated, it is important doctors are around to deal with anything unexpected. "

3. **What do you think most people who qualify in medicine do?**

Despite most people associating medicine with the hospital environment, the reality is that up to 50% of doctors are actually GPs. If you didn't know that before, its a good time to learn it.

The reason for most doctors being GPs is that the majority of people access healthcare though their GP, who would either deal with their problem there, or refer to a hospital specialist. As this only leaves around 50% of positions left to become surgeons and physicians across a multitude specialities, it means that these specialities are often very competitive to get into.

"Although medicine for me, has always been associated with hospital medicine, I found out recently on the GMC register that nearly 30% of doctors are fully qualified GPs on the GP register, making it the largest single speciality and with many more who will still be in GP

training. Although it is surprising, it does make

sense as most individuals with illness have long

term problems which the GP can deal with."

4. Have you ever considered becoming a G.P.?

As above with such a high percentage of
doctors becoming GPs, it would be wise to
consider it as a career path. Although it may not
seem as glamorous as hospital medicine, this is
where you as a doctor can make a lasting
positive effect on a community, as well as
building the best patient-doctor relationships.
With a more flexible training pathway and
reliable job hours, it offers freedom compared
to some other medical career pathways. With
the opportunity to become a special interest

GP, you can find yourself a niche within general practice. Furthermore, with the introduction of the NHS white paper, it is more likely that GPs will be instrumental in shaping the future of the NHS.

"I hadn't considered being a GP before, mainly because I have always thought that I would find surgery much more interesting as a career path, however, I can see that it has some great benefits as a possible career choice and to be honest, during my time researching more into areas of medicine, I think I would like to keep an open mind to other career choices and would want to wait until I have experienced some clinical medicine before I make my final decision on where I want to be."

5. What are the positive and negative aspects about being a doctor?

Like any career, there will always be positive sand negatives of the job and it is whether those positives outweigh the negatives that makes the career worthwhile for you. Being a doctor is a privileged position where you are privy to the most private parts of human existence, dealing with people at their most vulnerable. It is well respected, provides great job satisfaction and is a secure job in most instances with decent pay, assuring a future in medicine.

However, medicine is still considered a vocation and there are many sacrifices to be made in becoming a doctor. Firstly, the length of course ranges from 5-6 years and therefore, one must has the determination and ambition to succeed. Secondly, particularly as a junior doctor the hours can be long and the climb to the top can be difficult, especially now that consultant posts are no longer guaranteed.

"Just like any job, being a doctor has its positives and negatives, however, for me the positives definitely outweigh the negative aspects of the job. Although the long unsociable hours and the length of the undergraduate course and further training may deter many

students, I believe that medicine has a lot to offer me. It is the chance to make a difference in people's lives every day by dealing with their health. Furthermore, it is still a well respected and well paid profession and I would love the opportunity to count myself in the same profession as some of the greatest innovators and pioneers of our world today."

6. Would you like to be a nurse?

Nurses are invaluable to the jobs that doctors do. They are responsible for the care which a patient receives on the wards, ensuring that they are closely monitored, drugs are administered correctly, while providing the personal care plans needed for a patient to recover from an illness. A common mistake which people often make when asked why they want to be a doctor is that they would like to care for people, which is the main role of a nurse. A doctor is responsible for managing a patient's care, but also for diagnosing, treating and preventing disease. It is important to make the distinction between the roles.

"The reason why I applied for medical school is because I want to be involved in finding a solution to a patient's health problem. I would like to be able to apply my scientific knowledge to deal with clinical situations and inevitably lead the healthcare team to deliver the best possible care as opposed to just administering

care. While I think nurses are invaluable to the job that doctors do, I believe that I can apply myself adequately to fulfil the role of a doctor."

7. Do you think a doctor's job is stressful?

A doctor's job can be stressful, if not more than most professions, and this is due to the sensitive nature of their work. Dealing with life and death on the daily basis is not a responsibility taken lightly and it puts added pressure on the decisions which need to be made regarding a patient's care. It has been known for a long time that doctors have one of the highest suicide rates and alcoholism compared to other professions and this is partly due to the stress that they feel they are under.

Use your work experience if possible to highlight a stressful situation.

"I think that doctor's are under a lot of stress as the decisions which they take on a daily basis can affect people's lives positively or negatively. Whilst on work experience, I witnessed doctors having to make difficult decisions about whether patients were well enough to be kept alive using drug treatment or whether they should be allowed to end their life more peacefully. Taking a decision like that cannot have been easy, particularly when some of the family members didn't agree with the decision. This is what adds to the stress of an already busy and demanding job, and I can understand

why the medical profession has a notorious reputation with alcohol abuse and suicide. It is for this reason, I believe that it is important to develop techniques for dealing with stress from the start."

8. **If you did not get onto the medicine course, what other profession would you be interested in?**

Medicine is one of the most competitive courses to study at university and it receives the highest number of applications. There is a greater chance of being denied a place at medical school than succeeding so you must be prepared and think about what you would do if your application this year was unsuccessful.

Although you may have wanted to do medicine all your life, try to use a question like this to re-evaluate your life. Think about the skills you have and how you could apply them or excel in any other professions, but end your answer re-affirming your desire to do medicine and describe how it is the only profession best suited to you.

"If I didn't get onto the medicine course, I would definitely take a gap year and re-apply. I believe that medicine is the career path which I want to take. In my gap year, I would improve my skills, gain more experience and insight and portray my dedication to this career choice. I do not have an alternative career choice in mind at the

moment, but I think that I would make a good mathematician as I have a very logical mind and Maths is one of my favourite subjects at AS level."

9. **What makes a good team member?**

Teamwork is essential in the healthcare setting and being a good team member is vital for ensuring the team operates at its highest level possible.

Attributes of a good team member:

- Not complacent

- Does not exert their own ego

- An effective communicator

- Willing to listen to others opinion

- Able to give and receive constructive criticism

- Contributes to team discussion and effort
- Works hard to ensure the goals of the team are met
- Puts the needs of their team above personal desires

These are just some of a few attributes of which a good team member is seen to have, with the most important being that you are willing to be cooperative with your team's efforts regardless of relationships within the team. Feel free to highlight examples of when you have been a good team member or some of the things which you have done to improve yourself and productivity within your team.

"I believe that being a good team member is

essential in the healthcare profession and in all walks of life where a group of people are needed to achieve a common goal. As part of my school football team, I have had the experience of seeing what helps make a good team player, with many of our team being great examples, which has been part of the reason for our recent cup successes. I think a good team member works hard for the team regardless of their position, is able to share in the responsibility of the team, both in its success and failure, and is able to communicate well in order to make sure everyone around them knows what is going on. I know that my experience of being a part of my school football team has allowed me to understand what a good team player is and I hope that it will stand

me in good stead for a future in medicine."

10. What qualities does a doctor need?

A study published by the Mayo Clinic in 2006 identified 7 traits which patients believed made a good doctor. These were:

- Confidence – a confident doctor inspires confidence from the patient

- Empathy – trying to understand what the patient is feeling and experiencing

- Humanity – being caring, compassionate and kind

- Being personal – being interested in the patient as an individual

- Forthright – talking to the patient honestly in everyday language

- Respect – taking into consideration a patients wishes and opinion

- Thorough – Being conscientious and persistent in looking after the patient

These are but a few of the characteristics of being a good doctor and what all doctors should be aspiring to be. The GMC offers great guidelines on what the duties and qualities of the doctor are in their Good Medical Practice section of their website: www.gmc-uk.org

You can use just a few of these attributes to answer the question. No one will be expecting you to reel off every positive trait thought to make up what a doctor should be or need.

"Having read the GMC guidelines on the duties of a doctor, I think that a doctor needs to have a number of qualities in order to carry out their job to a basic level. Firstly they must be humane, being able to put the care of their patients at the forefront of decision making. Doctors must be respectful, and be able to work with the patient, taking into consideration their wishes and opinions. Finally, they should be honest and act with integrity in order to both ensure that the patient understands what is going on, and to ensure that they do not discriminate as part of their job."

11. A banker works long hours, why are they different from a doctor?

A banker and doctor are similar in that they both make decisions over sensitive aspects of people's lives, their money and their health. However, the job descriptions of the two are very different and the trust placed in the two roles are different. This leads to greater pressure on doctors as they are often under more personal responsibility for their actions. Furthermore, the interests of doctors and bankers are very different. A banker's sole interest is to ensure the profits for their bank, whereas a doctor is bound to put the concerns of their patients first, this means that patients are able to trust doctors more in their decisions than clients are of bankers. This is acceptable and fair, however, because of this trust, if anything was to go wrong with a procedure it means that the doctor is more personally responsible, whereas if something went wrong with a bank deal, bankers are often absolved of the responsibility by passing the risks onto the customer by default. It is in this personal responsibility which makes the long hours worked by doctors much more difficult than those worked by bankers regardless of workload.

"Even though both doctors and banker work long hours, the difference lies in the level of responsibility that is assumed each time they are expected to work. While bankers can be

absolved of their actions by passing all risks back to their customers, doctors can only do that in part. If a decision made by a doctor is found to be wrong, regardless of whether the risks were informed, that doctor is still responsible for the mistake that he made, and could be made liable for them. This is the main reason why doctors are required to have indemnity insurance."

NHS 2013 changes based questions

We will keep this chapter short and concise. When you invited to a medical school interviews it is unlikely that you will be asked complex or detailed questions about the National Health Service (NHS). This knowledge will develop over your undergraduate training and after graduation in in your foundation training year. In our advice, we do not ask you to try and learn everything possible about practicing medicine within the

NHS; there is a lot and it can be confusing. Focus on understanding the main principles, recent changes, mechanisms and payment options, in order to be able to answer the standard questions that will be asked.

Some of this has been covered in other chapters but we will discuss the background of the NHS, a few successes and failures and what the future holds. This should give you enough material to evaluate, critique and comment upon during your interview.

The NHS was founded on July 5th 1948 by Aneurin Bevan, the Health Secretary at the time. His plan was to, for the first time, bring hospitals, doctors, nurses, pharmacists, opticians and dentists together under one umbrella organisation to provide services that are free for all at the point of delivery.

Aneurin believed good healthcare should be accessible to all, regardless of wealth, a core principle which has been upheld to this day. Healthcare is financed entirely from taxation, which means that people pay according to what is feasible for them. The NHS is the largest publicly funded health service in the world. However, there are three services that are not free at the point of delivery. They are:

1. Prescriptions

2. Optical services

3. Dental Services

There is a yearly NHS budget which is allocated at calculated percentages to all the different fields. For 2012 to 2013, this budget was set by the Parliament at £108.9 billion. You can look online for the percentage breakdown if this is interests you but it is unlikely that you will asked this in an interview.

A useful website to use at this stage is the NHS Choices website which outlines the NHS, its set up, principles and treatments available for the general public. It concisely and explains everything and may help answer any questions you have.

Previously all NHS planning and delivery was implemented by The Department of Health

(DOH), strategic health authorities (SHAs) and primary care trusts (PCTs). The secretary for state of health (Jeremy Hunt) oversaw all major decisions and reported directly to the Prime Minister.

As of 2013, the NHS is being re-vamped per say and as per such is going through a number of changes within its core structure. Most of these changes recently took effect on April 1, 2013.

The changes are keeping in accordance with the Health and Social Care Bill proposed by Andrew Lansley in 2012. Therefore, some organisations such as the aforementioned PCTs and SHAs will be gradually abolished and in its place will enter new organisations such as clinical commissioning groups (CCGs). Furthermore, local authorities will have more responsibilities for budgets relating to public health. It is important that you understand that there are a wide range of NHS health trusts which are involved in managing NHS hospital care in England, including community care and mental health services. All of these NHS trusts are to become foundation trusts by 2014. You can find detailed information about the individual trusts and upcoming changes on the NHS choices website.

A summary of the Health and Social Care Bill, 2012 (www.parliament.co.uk):

The Bill proposes to create an independent NHS Board, promote patient choice, and to reduce

NHS administration costs.

Key areas that will be affected:

- An independent NHS Board will be established to allocate resources and provide commissioning guidance

- GPs' will have more power to commission services on behalf of their patients

- The role of the Care Quality Commission will be fortified

- A new body called Monitor will be created. This will convert the body that currently regulates NHS foundation trusts, into an economic regulator to oversee aspects of access and competition in the NHS

- In order to cut NHS administration costs by a third, a number of health bodies will be abolished, including abolishing Primary Care Trusts and Strategic Health Authorities.

Although all these changes have started to take effect, their impact on the public will be gradual and it is important that you have a general understanding of which bodies are to be abolished and which new ones will take their place. This should be sufficient with respect to your interview preparation.

1. Can patients receive any treatment they want under the NHS?

"The DOH states that 'any individual who normally resides in the UK is entitled to free NHS hospital treatment in England, whereas anyone who is not ordinarily a resident, is subject to the NHS (charges to overseas visitors)'. Although this is the case, there are certain treatments which are free to all which includes any treatment given in an accident and emergency (A & E) department, certain treatments provided by a walk-in centre, treatment for certain communicable diseases, imperative psychiatric treatment and family planning services. Meanwhile prescriptions, optical services and dental services are not provided free of charge. "

2. If the NHS is funded by taxation and patients need to pay for dental treatment, what happens to those patients who are not currently being taxed?

"In these situations there are certain 'exemptions' or 'allowances' made for these patients. The following patients will not need to pay for treatment at the point of delivery:

▶ *Anyone aged under 18*

▶ *Anyone under 19 and receiving full-time education*

▶ *Anyone pregnant or has had a baby in the previous 12 months*

- *Anyone staying in an NHS hospital and the treatment is carried out by the hospital dentist*
- *An NHS hospital dental service outpatient (however, you may have to pay for your dentures or bridges)*
- *Anyone on Income Support*
- *Anyone on Income-related Employment and Support Allowance*
- *Anyone on Income-based Jobseeker's Allowance*
- *Anyone on Pension Credit guarantee credit*
- *If you are named on a valid NHS tax credit exemption certificate or you are*

entitled to an NHS tax credit

exemption certificate"

3. **On your application I can see that you did some work experience in a GP clinic and on an acute ward in a hospital. What differences did you observe and which did you prefer?**

The NHS primary care is defined as your first point of contact with the health services, so this would be your GP or a walk in centre or any emergency services. Secondary care is care provided for you in a hospital setting by a specialist. Lastly, tertiary care is further specialist treatment in a hospital.

There are some apparent differences when comparing both work settings. A working doctor in a hospital is required to work cohesively in a multi- disciplinary team, whereby there are usual inter-disciplinary meetings (involving doctors, nurses, physiotherapists etc.), handovers and a routine of opinion seeking from seniors. In a GP clinic, the doctor is the sole decision maker and depending on the history and clinical examination of the patient, they need to decipher whether the respective patient requires urgent care, or can be given a prescription and asked to return at a later date.

"It was really eye-opening to witness first-hand, the care with which the GP conveyed sensitive information to his patients but also how

important communication was on a whole, particularly for patients in the community where English is not their first language. Meanwhile, in the busy acute ward it was interesting to observe the faster paced routine of a doctor, especially during ward rounds as they moved from one patient to the next, emphasising the importance of time management and empathy."

4. **Can you give an example of any recent unsuccessful ventures undertaken by the NHS? Why do you think it was unsuccessful?**

This is where you can score bonus points and show the interviewer that you have a good understanding of current affairs associated with the NHS. Make sure that you always weigh up your answers and do not just emphasise on the negative aspects of the given situation.

One good example is that of NPFIT (National Programme for IT), which was launched in 2004. It was launched with the aim to integrate all IT systems within the NHS in order to improve delivery of care. This included providing high speed broadband service, electronic records, an NHS number for every new born baby, choose and book etc. However, the initial allocated budget spiraled out of control and the project was scrapped a couple of years later, costing the NHS billions!

"I remember reading about the government's

project- NPFIT, where although the initial aims were ambitious and purposeful, the lack of managers involving clinicians in decisions led to problems. I found it interesting to learn that when it came down to implementing various parts of the programme, there was resistance from members of staff at pretty much all levels of care. This highlights the importance of involving all parties in any major transformative decision, particularly in healthcare where teamwork and co-operation is of utmost importance, in order to deliver the best care"

5. **Can you give an example of any projects undertaken by the NHS that have been a success?**

Once again you can use this type of a question to elaborate on recent events within the NHS. The best way to do this is by keeping up to date with the news, the official NHS website (www.nhs.uk) and other related articles.

One such example is NHS direct which was launched in 1998 after the government identified the need for a telephone service. The service itself became active in the year 2000; accessibility 24 hours a day, 7 days a week all year round make it unique and successful. This was later followed by a phone app (which is now available on all smart phones). The site has an application called symptom checker which helps to filter urgent cases from the not so serious ones. This has helped to enormously reduce patients unnecessarily visiting their GPs and saved the NHS money which could potentially be used elsewhere. All in all NHS direct has helped to save the NHS millions spent per year.

"With the NHS being run on such a tight budget, it is crucial that any successful venture delivers cost savings, one prime example being that of NHS direct. Although this was launched over a decade ago, it continues to save the NHS money and has further transpired into newer forms of technology such as mobile apps etc. Monetary savings form one part of the picture whilst other advances such as the PACS (picture archiving and communication system) delivers efficiency and improved quality in the provision of care for patients. Whilst working on the wards I

remember seeing doctors use the PACS system to view X-rays, CT scans and MRIs during ward rounds. This is a leading example of how advances in technology have benefited patient care."

6. **Do you know of any upcoming advances in healthcare that the NHS is supporting?**

Developed countries such as that of the UK knowingly have an increased burden of chronic illnesses (such as diabetes and heart disease) alongside an increasingly ageing population. With these changes in society, the face of healthcare delivery has altered from the once known eradication of life threatening illnesses to now treating diseases that have resulted from obesity, smoking and other developments in society. Therefore, a lot of advances now involve ways to better care for the elderly and means to improve the quality of life of patients with chronic illnesses.

A good example to discuss here would be Telehealth; whereby with the use of telecommunications to continuously monitor patients, you reduce the frequency of them visiting their doctor. This gives patients more independence and confidence in managing their own condition whilst saving the NHS money. Devices include monitors that update important information about the patient and send it straight to the GP, such as their blood pressure, blood sugar levels etc. Similarly, Telecare is another facet where the potential use of technology can help elderly patients live a more independent and whole life. This is of great value to patients with cognitive impairment or forms of dementia and includes devices that ease their day to day life. For instance, a remote control that enables them to open their front door from the living room, and a tracker that will alert local services if they ever get lost etc.

With any new advances, remember to do the research to back its claims and if you use an example, make sure you can actually back it up with evidence from a journal or scientific paper that you have read. By doing so, your argument will look a lot more robust. This will portray your ability to critically think and analyse given information.

7. What do you know about the General Medical Council?

The General Medical Council or the GMC is the body responsible to regulate doctors, ensuring that they are fit to practice in order to ensure good medical practice. Their primary purpose is to:

"protect, promote and maintain the health and safety of the public by ensuring proper standards in the practice of medicine"- www.gmc-uk.org

Please visit the official website, www.gmc-uk.org to understand their roles and responsibilities further. Doctors who practice in the UK, must be registered by the GMC and are given a GMC number.

"The GMC has four main functions based upon the Medical Act 1983 (www.gmc-uk.org):

- keeping up-to-date registers of qualified doctors
- nurturing good medical practice
- promoting high standards of medical education and training
- dealing firmly and fairly with doctors whose fitness to practice is in question.

8. Do you know the purpose of the British Medical Association?

The British Medical Association or the BMA is a

trusted body that represents doctors both locally and nationally. The representative body is made up of 560 doctors from all parts of the profession who meet at the annual representative meeting (ARM) to vote and decide on key issues. The BMA also provides support and help to students and doctors that are undergoing training. Practical support that they provide include aspects of guidance and help on redundancies, pensions, ethical concerns, whistle blowing, European Working Time directive rules etc.

Please visit www.bma.org.uk for a detailed understanding of their roles and responsibilities.

"The BMA is a trusted body that provides support and help in the form of advice, guidance

and free resources for medical students and graduate doctors. They are at the forefront of fighting for doctors' rights and help doctors throughout their training process all the way from foundation training to specialities."

9. If you could change one thing about the NHS what would it be and why?

This is a difficult question as there is no one correct answer. We encourage you to be confident in what you say and make your answer personal based on either your work experience, or on your ideals for a 'perfect NHS'. This will enable the interviewer to see your personality through your choice of answer. Remember the key issues that the NHS is constantly scrutinised for – the lack of resources (money, staff and equipment) to meet the ever-growing demand (increasing number of patients using NHS services). Ideally, you should answer this keeping these issues in mind.

"Due to the free provision of healthcare, I believe that there is a tendency for people to misuse and abuse the system, for example by missing appointments over and over and by not adhering to their medication regime etc. To improve things, I would suggest charging the public a minimal fee for using any service provided by the NHS. In this way they may be more prone to be accountable for their actions and will think twice about wasting resources. It is interesting that France has the world's best healthcare and all

patients there have to pay the entire amount of the service they require upfront, even though a majority of it gets refunded back to them. This nonetheless makes them aware of how expensive things actually are and if an aspect like that was introduced here in the UK, it would translate in to huge cost savings for the NHS."

20266

11246110R00180

Printed in Great Britain
by Amazon.co.uk, Ltd.,
Marston Gate.